Commonsense Nutrition

A Guide to Good Health for Your Family

Commonsense Nutrition

A Guide to Good Health for Your Family

by Ruth Little Carey, Ph.D.
Irma Bachmann Vyhmeister, M.S.
Jennie Stagg Hudson, M.A.

Pacific Press Publishing Association
Mountain View, California; Omaha, Nebraska
Oshawa, Ontario

Dedicated to the students who through
the years added interest, zest, and challenge
to the School of Nutrition and Dietetics
of Loma Linda University.

Reprinted 1975, 1976, 1978

Library of Congress Catalog Card No. 77-142796

Acknowledgments

Acknowledgments are sincerely made to Alice Garrett Marsh, M.S., professor of home economics, Andrews University, for critical reading of a previous draft; and to the following from Loma Linda University School of Nutrition and Dietetics: Florence Tidwell Otto, M.S., instructor, for work on an early draft of the book; Barbara Jemison Myer, M.S., assistant professor, for reading and suggestions; Vera Mae Marsh Hanson, M.S., assistant professor, and her Special Problems Class (Rose Budd Ludlow, Selma Chaij Lukens, Annie Cristobel Stubblefield, Daysi Cunningham, Marian Fedak, Georgia Hodgkin, Judith Lampy, Linda Schultz, Wilmer Snyder, and Ellen Velasco Martin) for their involvement in some preliminary work.

This book was prepared by the School of Nutrition and Dietetics of Loma Linda University as a scientific nutrition source book with the sincere hope that it would prove of value to many individuals.

The Authors

Contents

Introduction

This book is designed as an easy-to-follow guide to good nutrition for the average layman, particularly the modern homemaker. For the homemaker, nutrition can be a very practical science, making possible longer lives and better health for everyone in the family. By applying the principles of good nutrition as she plans and prepares meals, today's homemaker can help her family members be healthier, more attractive people. Her children benefit from stronger teeth and bones, clearer complexions, and higher resistance to troublesome colds and viruses. Her husband is in better condition to avoid crippling and sometimes murderous heart disease, and she enjoys a trimmer figure. Even Grandma and Grandpa can be better prepared physically and emotionally to enjoy their retirement years by applying the basic principles of nutrition to their diet. All of these subjects and more are covered in *Commonsense Nutrition.*

The homemaker will also be happy to find such useful subjects as how to satisfy a teen-age appetite; tips for packing tasty, attractive sack lunches; and how to handle a salt-free diet. The chapter titled "Can a Vegetarian Be Healthy?" along with several vegetarian menus featured in other chapters, will especially interest those who prefer to serve their family a vegetarian diet. The many meal plans and suggested menus provide a special bonus. Recipes for most of the entrées and special dishes listed can be found in *Vegetarian Cookery,* the five-volume cookbook series also published by Pacific Press.

A confusing array of nutritional data flowing regularly from field and research laboratories confronts anyone who proposes to organize a practical volume on nutrition. But the highly qualified professionals who sorted and selected the material for this book somehow condensed the mass of facts into a readable, well-organized guide to good nutrition—and all in the language of the layman. The three authors, each of them a professor of nutrition, are accustomed to translating the language of science into language understandable to students. The work was done under the direction of Ruth Little Carey, Ph.D., former director of the School of Nutrition and Dietetics at Loma Linda University in southern California.

The Editors

Nutrition Concerns You Too

The human machine which forms our body must be fueled regularly with food. Thus an understanding of nutrition—the science concerned with the function and bodily assimilation of this food fuel—is essential to ensure healthy, active lives for ourselves and our families. Nutrition involves every facet of our lives. It affects our spiritual and mental development as well as our physical well-being. Our whole life—our very existence, health, and ability to work and contribute to the society in which we live—depends upon adequate nutrition.

Nutrition involves food, the nutrients food contains, and the functions and requirements of these nutrients within the body. Man has always recognized the importance of food to his health and survival. In fact, the first known professions—farming, shepherding, and hunting—were related to food, or, in other words, to nutrition.

The greatest problems facing the world today involve the elimination of malnutrition—the provision of adequate nutrition. Consider, for example, the case of ten-year-old Johnny.

One day a teacher found Johnny sitting on the stairs of the schoolhouse, staring at the floor.

"What's wrong, Johnny? Shouldn't you be in class?" the teacher asked.

"I don't know."

"What are you doing here then?"

"Nothing."

Something in his pale face told her that Johnny's problem might not be a disciplinary one. He clenched his fists and held his arms tight against his lean body. He looked small and subdued.

A disturbing thought crossed the teacher's mind. "Did you have breakfast this morning, Johnny?"

"Ye-s-s," came his slow and uncertain reply.

"What did you eat?" she asked.

"Coffee."

"And for lunch?"

He did not answer. For a second his eyes flickered; then he hunched down to his original position.

"You did not have any lunch?"

He blinked. Then he fixed his eyes on her. "There was no food left," he whispered.

She looked at his pale face, his meager body, his defeated attitude; then she handed him a permission slip to get some food from the lunch room. This food would alleviate his hunger, but only temporarily.

Johnny's problem is not unique. Millions of the people of the world today never know what it is not to be hungry. More than half the world's population of three billion, according to reports, are malnourished. But these are just statistics. It is impossible to comprehend a billion men, women, and children, or even a million. Johnny's teacher became acutely aware of hunger because she actually saw it. Can you visualize those malnourished millions as real children and living adults with feelings of comfort or pain, of satisfaction or gnawing hunger?

In contrast to the hungry and starving millions, there are those who have enough food, frequently too much, but who do not choose the right kind. They, too, are malnourished. Whether one is hungry or overfed, nutrition in one way or another concerns everyone.

The ultimate goal of nutrition is buoyant health. But how can millions like Johnny throughout the world be healthy without sufficient food? How can sufficient food be supplied to them? On the other side, how can those who have access to large amounts of food be taught and motivated to choose wisely for good nutrition? These are the problems of nutrition, your problems as well as problems of the experts.

Organizations and individuals around the world work earnestly to fulfill the urgent need to provide food and eradicate hunger and malnutrition. A lecturer at the seventy-first Congress of American Industry stated that "balancing food production with consumption requirements is truly global. . . . Man's quest for peace—our very survival—may well rest on achieving this balance."

The task is not easy. The fact is, it seems almost impossible. Aside from all of the formidable intricacies of producing and transporting ample nutrients, there are racial, social, and psychological influences connected with food.

Food habits, for example, are ingrained in each person. They are a personal matter, attached to cultural patterns and sense of values. Even children have an innate resistance to changing their food habits. Persuading people to accept new types of food is a big problem in overcoming malnutrition. Americans working for the Government discover this time and again when trying to bring relief to famine areas. No matter how tasty or nutritious a food, if people will not eat it, it is useless. Nutritionists have made it their study to adjust the pattern of an adequate diet to existing food habits.

In Johnny's case the nutrition problem involved real hunger, whereas in more prosperous lands such as most of North America, the problem is over gratification of appetite with the wrong foods. Then there are the psychological factors which affect nutrition. Food may mean relief from anxiety for the emotionally unstable; it may mean a link with the homeland and a sense of security for the immigrant; advancing socially for the socialite; pleasure for the gourmet. In the family circle, food means more than the provision of adequate nutrients, more than the satisfaction of appetite. It expresses love, goodwill, friendship, and hospitality. It is often at the family table that personal ties become stronger, and mental, physical, spiritual, and social well-being are enhanced.

Adequate nutrition is essential at each stage of life from the tiny infant to the great-grandparent. Each period of life has special stresses and needs.

Research has shown that malnutrition during the first few years of life not only produces a sickly baby, but affects health and even mentality in later life. Some specialists believe that the critical period in the development of the brain and central nervous system comes during the last three months of fetus and the first two years of life.

There is growing evidence that malnutrition during these important periods can cause irreversible physical and mental damage. Another important aspect of nutrition is its effect upon infection. Good nutrition tends to prevent infections by aiding the normal operation of the body's defense mechanisms.

It has been shown that nutrition may affect our disposition and appearance. Research also points the finger at nutrition in connection with length of life, intelligence, learning, memory, and prevention of senility, all of these matters being of particular concern in the adult years.

How can the goal of adequate nutrition for everyone be accomplished? Much scientific information, such as the Recommended Daily Dietary Allowances of the National Research Council,* has become available through nutritional research, surveys, and field work. Can this information be useful to us in a personal way?

First, this information must be translated into a language understood by all, and this language is foods. To be told to drink half a glass of orange juice daily for vitamin C needs is far more meaningful for the average person than to be told the specified milligrams of ascorbic acid required. Three cups of milk as a daily requirement is much simpler to understand than 800 milligrams of calcium. In the language of food, nutritional information becomes simple and can be understood by nearly everyone.

Second, this information must be channeled into practical guides for meal planning. Our grandmothers guessed at the needs of their families. Some guessed quite well, but many guessed wrong. Today choosing an adequate diet requires no guesswork. Scientific guides are available to indicate the foods necessary for good nutrition. The best known of these guides is the "Four Food Groups" which gives much information without being technical. A homemaker can follow the Four Food Groups guide and be assured, under normal conditions, of a well-fed family. Furthermore, these guides are flexible and can be adapted to the food supplies in other lands.

Third, nutrition must be related to health. Remember that health does not refer to the physical aspect of life only. It involves more than

---

*The 1968 revision of the National Research Council (NRC) Recommended Daily Dietary Allowances (RDA) is based on current research and is a guide to nutrient needs for healthy individuals in the United States. See pages 16, 17.

that, encompassing all of you—your physical, mental, spiritual, and social well-being.

Knowledge of nutrition has brought hope for a better life even for those in diseased conditions. The success of the modern diabetic in enjoying a normal life, by intelligent management of his diet, activity, and insulin, is a far cry from the former situation in which the diabetic had no hope.

The length of our life and our freedom from disease center around good nutrition. By choosing our food wisely we can help our body and mind to remain active and useful. Adequate nutrition means hope and fulfillment, better health and greater vigor for everyone, including our own families and all the Johnnys around the world.

The floodlight of modern research is helping people "to understand how much their habits of diet have to do with their health, their characters, their usefulness in this world, and their eternal destiny." —Ellen G. White, *Testimonies,* Vol. 1, pp. 488, 489.

Food and Nutrition Board, National Academy of Sciences—National Research Council
RECOMMENDED DAILY DIETARY ALLOWANCES,[a] Revised 1968
Designed for the maintenance of good nutrition of practically all healthy people in the U.S.A

	Age[b] (years) From–To	Weight (kg)	Weight (lbs)	Height cm	Height (in)	kcal	Protein (gm)	Fat-Soluble Vitamins: Vitamin A Activity (IU)	Vitamin D (IU)	Vitamin E Activi (IU)
Infants	0-1/6	4	9	55	22	kgX120	kgX2.2[e]	1,500	400	5
	1/6-1/2	7	15	63	25	kgX110	kgX2.0[e]	1,500	400	5
	1/2-1	9	20	72	28	kgX100	kgX1.8[e]	1,500	400	5
Children	1-2	12	26	81	32	1,100	25	2,000	400	10
	2-3	14	31	91	36	1,250	25	2,000	400	10
	3-4	16	35	100	39	1,400	30	2,500	400	10
	4-6	19	42	110	43	1,600	30	2,500	400	10
	6-8	23	51	121	48	2,000	35	3,500	400	15
	8-10	28	62	131	52	2,200	40	3,500	400	15
Males	10-12	35	77	140	55	2,500	45	4,500	400	20
	12-14	43	95	151	59	2,700	50	5,000	400	20
	14-18	59	130	170	67	3,000	60	5,000	400	25
	18-22	67	147	175	69	2,800	60	5,000	400	30
	22-35	70	154	175	69	2,800	65	5,000	—	30
	35-55	70	154	173	68	2,600	65	5,000	—	30
	55-75+	70	154	171	67	2,400	65	5,000	—	30
Females	10-12	35	77	142	56	2,250	50	4,500	400	20
	12-14	44	97	154	61	2,300	50	5,000	400	20
	14-16	52	114	157	62	2,400	55	5,000	400	25
	16-18	54	119	160	63	2,300	55	5,000	400	25
	18-22	58	128	163	64	2,000	55	5,000	400	25
	22-35	58	128	163	64	2,000	55	5,000	—	25
	35-55	58	128	160	63	1,850	55	5,000	—	25
	55-75+	58	128	157	62	1,700	55	5,000	—	25
Pregnancy						+200	65	6,000	400	30
Lactation						+1,000	75	8,000	400	30

[a] The allowance levels are intended to cover individual variations among most normal persons as they live in the United States under usual environmental stresses. The recommended allowances can be attained with a variety of common foods, providing other nutrients for which human requirements have been less well defined. See text for more-detailed discussion of allowances and of nutrients not tabulated.

[b] Entries on lines for age range 22-35 years represent the reference man and woman at age 22. All other entries represent allowances for the midpoint of the specified age range.

Water-Soluble Vitamins							Minerals				
Ascorbic Acid (mg)	Folacin[c] (mg)	Niacin (mg equiv)[d]	Riboflavin (mg)	Thiamin (mg)	Vitamin B_6 (mg)	Vitamin B_{12} (mg)	Calcium (g)	Phosphorus (g)	Iodine (mg)	Iron (mg)	Magnesium (mg)
35	0.05	5	0.4	0.2	0.2	1.0	0.4	0.2	25	6	40
35	0.05	7	0.5	0.4	0.3	1.5	0.5	0.4	40	10	60
35	0.1	8	0.6	0.5	0.4	2.0	0.6	0.5	45	15	70
40	0.1	8	0.6	0.6	0.5	2.0	0.7	0.7	55	15	100
40	0.2	8	0.7	0.6	0.6	2.5	0.8	0.8	60	15	150
40	0.2	9	0.8	0.7	0.7	3	0.8	0.8	70	10	200
40	0.2	11	0.9	0.8	0.9	4	0.8	0.8	80	10	200
40	0.2	13	1.1	1.0	1.0	4	0.9	0.9	100	10	250
40	0.3	15	1.2	1.1	1.2	5	1.0	1.0	110	10	250
40	0.4	17	1.3	1.3	1.4	5	1.2	1.2	125	10	300
45	0.4	18	1.4	1.4	1.6	5	1.4	1.4	135	18	350
55	0.4	20	1.5	1.5	1.8	5	1.4	1.4	150	18	400
60	0.4	18	1.6	1.4	2.0	5	0.8	0.8	140	10	400
60	0.4	18	1.7	1.4	2.0	5	0.8	0.8	140	10	350
60	0.4	17	1.7	1.3	2.0	5	0.8	0.8	125	10	350
60	0.4	14	1.7	1.2	2.0	6	0.8	0.8	110	10	350
40	0.4	15	1.3	1.1	1.4	5	1.2	1.2	110	18	300
45	0.4	15	1.4	1.2	1.6	5	1.3	1.3	115	18	350
50	0.4	16	1.4	1.2	1.8	5	1.3	1.3	120	18	350
50	0.4	15	1.5	1.2	2.0	5	1.3	1.3	115	18	350
55	0.4	13	1.5	1.0	2.0	5	0.8	0.8	100	18	350
55	0.4	13	1.5	1.0	2.0	5	0.8	0.8	100	18	300
55	0.4	13	1.5	1.0	2.0	5	0.8	0.8	90	18	300
55	0.4	13	1.5	1.0	2.0	6	0.8	0.8	80	10	300
60	0.8	15	1.8	+0.1	2.5	8	+0.4	+0.4	125	18	450
60	0.5	20	2.0	+0.5	2.5	6	+0.5	+0.5	150	18	450

[c] The folacin allowances refer to dietary sources as determined by ***Lactobacillus casei*** assay. Pure forms of folacin may be effective in doses less than ¼ of the RDA.
[d] Niacin equivalents include dietary sources of the vitamin itself plus 1 mg equivalent for each 60 mg of dietary tryptophan.
[e] Assumes protein equivalent to human milk. For proteins not 100 percent utilized factors should be increased proportionately.

A Daily Food Guide

"What Shall We Eat?" is the title of an old cookbook with a copyright date of 1868. The title page states that it is "A Manual for Housekeepers, comprising a bill of fare for breakfast, dinner, and tea for every day in the year." The preface further states that "The design of this manual is to suggest to ladies, without the trouble of thinking, what is seasonable for the table."

Like the old cookbook, a modern daily food guide helps you answer the question "What shall we eat?" but unlike the cookbook it is not intended to aid you "without the trouble of *thinking.*" Rather, it assists you in thinking and offers a pattern that should make choosing good, nutritious meals for your family easier.

The Daily Food Guide is an interpretation in common foods of the National Research Council Recommended Daily Dietary Allowances (RDA).* It recommends adequate daily amounts of calories and protein, five minerals, and ten vitamins for men, women (including pregnant and nursing women), infants, and children at various ages. The minerals and vitamins which it omits either do not have an established human requirement or are so widely distributed in foods that they are seldom lacking in the diet if the other requirements are met.

A panel of nutrition experts determines the allowances according to current scientific findings. They allow for margins of safety above what are believed to be the minimum requirements of these nutrients. The allowances are designed for normally active, healthy persons

*See pages 16, 17 for 1968 revision.

living in a temperate climate such as the United States. In hotter or colder countries the needs for some of the nutrients vary. Nutritional needs increase during pregnancy and lactation and vary during childhood and adolescence. Illness also affects the requirements.

The Daily Food Guide differs from the RDA. It offers a framework for nutritious meals. It is not a complete menu, but consists of four food groups with suggested portions. In using the Guide, choose at least the minimum number of servings recommended from each group. Then select additional foods to round out the diet to maintain ideal weight.

Choose from day to day and week to week a wide variety of wholesome foods, because each food contributes not one but several essential nutrients. Variety is needed to ensure good nutrition.

DAILY FOOD GUIDE

1. Protein foods—2 servings or more from the following:
   Cheese, eggs, mature legumes, nuts, vegetable proteins either commercially or home prepared (such as gluten, soyameat, nutmeat, and cereal-legume-nut combinations of appreciable protein content), meat, including fowl and fish.
2. Milk and milk products:
   Children—2 to 4 cups
   Teen-agers—3 to 4 cups (boys may drink more)
   Adults—2 or more cups
3. Vegetables and fruits:
   4 or more servings
   Dark green or deep yellow vegetable at least every other day
   Leafy green vegetables freely
   Other vegetables, including potatoes, liberally
   Citrus fruit or juice, tomato juice or other foods high in vitamin C, daily
   Other fruits liberally
4. Breads and cereals:
   4 or more servings
   Whole grain, preferably; otherwise, enriched or restored

Fats as such are not mentioned in the Daily Food Guide although they are an essential part of the diet. The reason is that the average American tends to include ample, if not too much, fat in his diet.

With the amounts of butter, cream, and salad dressing customarily used in seasoning or on bread, and with that present in such foods as milk, eggs, nuts, olives, and avocados, there is little possibility of a deficiency. In general, fats from vegetable sources are to be preferred. They contain a higher percentage of essential polyunsaturatd fatty acids.

As we look more closely at the groups within the Guide we can see that each contributes to our daily needs.

The *protein group* has a variety of foods from which to choose. It is wise to use some protein food or milk product at each meal.

Cottage cheese is a good source of protein. Four ounces (one-half cup) furnishes 15 grams or approximately one-fourth of the day's requirement of protein. In the making of cottage cheese some calcium and riboflavin are separated in the whey, thus cottage cheese is lower in these two nutrients than milk. Cheddar type cheeses, if made from whole milk, contain similar properties to that of milk. One ounce of processed cheddar cheese contains calcium equal to two-thirds cup of milk.

Eggs supply about equal amounts of high quality protein and fat. They are a good source of vitamin A and iron and supply some riboflavin and thiamine and varying amounts of other minerals and vitamins. The yolk furnishes most of the minerals, vitamins, and fat. The fat is in a finely emulsified, easily digested form. Egg yolk is high in cholesterol. For this reason only three to four eggs a week are suggested.

Legumes are an inexpensive source of protein. When used simultaneously with other foods such as whole wheat they are of good nutritional value—high in starch, a good source of thiamine, niacin, and iron, and a fair source of calcium.

Soybeans or soy flour and chick-peas (garbanzos) are almost comparable to meat in protein value. Soybeans are a good source of iron and are higher in fat than other legumes.

Peanuts, legumes resembling nuts in texture and fat content, are one of the richest sources of niacin and a good source of protein. Four tablespoons of peanut butter supply about the same amount of protein as 2 ounces of lean cooked meat (without bone).

All nuts contain fair amounts of proteins. Unlike legumes, they contain little starch but are rich in fat. They contribute from fair to generous amounts of thiamine, riboflavin, and niacin, and good amounts of iron. Nuts and legumes deserve a large place in the diet and should be classed as protein-rich foods. Because nuts are compact in texture and high in fat, they should be chewed thoroughly and eaten in small amounts at a time, preferably with other foods.

Prepared vegetable proteins made of legumes, cereals (including wheat gluten), various forms of soybeans, and nuts, lend variety to your menu and are valuable sources of protein. Like nuts and legumes, their value is enhanced when served in combination with milk, eggs, and green, leafy vegetables. Products made from gluten, a wheat protein, may be used in planning diets low in fat and carbohydrate.

Milk and milk products are especially important for their high-quality protein, calcium, phosphorus, and riboflavin content. Milk is a good source of most of the essential nutrients but contains only small amounts of iron and vitamin C. It is of special value in the diets of growing children, adolescents, and pregnant and nursing women because it aids in building new tissues, bones, teeth, and muscles.

Some people prefer to substitute vegetable milk for cow's milk. They most commonly use soybean milk. It contains a good protein and some vitamins and minerals. Unless it is enriched, however, one half cup contains only 48 milligrams of calcium in contrast to the 118 milligrams in cow's milk. Although it has more than twice the thiamine of cow's milk, vegetable milk needs to be fortified with calcium and vitamin B_{12} if used as a substitute.

Vegetables and fruits are good sources of minerals and vitamins. Most of them do not contain much protein. The protein of green, leafy vegetables is of high quality, but is in too minute a quantity to make an appreciable contribution to the daily diet. Dark green leafy and deep yellow vegetables are excellent sources of carotene, which the body turns into vitamin A. Raw cabbage, broccoli, cauliflower, green peppers, and some other vegetables are good sources of vitamin C.

Potatoes, sweet potatoes, and yams are comparatively high in carbohydrate. Although not the best sources of vitamin C, they contribute good amounts of this vitamin and other minerals and vitamins. Sweet potatoes and yams, like other yellow vegetables, furnish carotene.

Other vegetables add variety to the diet and when used liberally add appreciable amounts of minerals and vitamins. They also improve greatly the general nutritional quality of the diet.

Fruits, because of their pleasing aroma, appearance, and flavor are a favorite food group. Citrus fruits and tomatoes contribute much of the vitamin C in the American diet. One cup of orange juice (canned, fresh, or frozen) will supply more than the day's requirement. The same amount of tomato juice supplies about half as much. Strawberries, papayas, and cantaloupes rate with citrus fruits in vitamin C content.

Deep yellow fruits such as persimmons, peaches, apricots, cantaloupes, and mangoes are excellent sources of carotene, the precursor of vitamin A. Dried fruits such as apricots, peaches, figs, dates, prunes, and raisins are concentrated sources of sugar, vitamins, and minerals, especially iron. Other fruits, including apples and bananas, add varying amounts of minerals and vitamins. When used plentifully, fruit makes the diet more palatable and nutritious.

Cereals and breads figure largely in the diets of many people of the world. They are rich in starch, and whole grain and enriched varieties contain valuable contributions of iron, thiamine, riboflavin, and niacin. When used liberally they also furnish substantial amounts of protein. Combined with milk, the protein is of high quality. Using a mixture of whole grains in cereals or breads increases the value of the protein.

Because the minerals and vitamins are held largely in the outer layers of the kernel or in the germ, most of them are lost in the milling process. Enriched or restored cereals and breads contain added thiamine, riboflavin, niacin, and iron. The practice of enrichment of white flour has helped many who use white bread and refined cereals. When possible it is better to choose largely from whole grain products and thus benefit from the additional nutrients they normally contain. You should note that the commonly found "wheat bread" (in contrast to 100% whole wheat bread) may contain less minerals and vitamins than enriched white bread.

Cellulose, or roughage, is the indigestible fiber found in whole grains, fruits, and vegetables. These foods, eaten in amounts suggested in the Daily Food Guide, furnish most of the roughage required in the diet and are desirable for the proper function of the digestive tract.

The chapter on menu planning which follows translates the Daily Food Guide into three meals a day.

In Summary

1. Choose daily from each food group at least the minimum amounts suggested in the Daily Food Guide.
2. Include a protein food or milk or both with each meal.
3. Choose a wide variety of wholesome, unrefined foods.
4. Eat enough to maintain ideal weight.

The Artist Within You: Menu Planning

Does the thought of planning a thousand menus stagger you? Many homemakers prepare and serve more than a thousand meals and snacks every year! Fortunately the meals usually come spaced at about three a day, but planning them can still be a chore. We hear frequent complaints from weary homemakers.

"I wish I knew what to fix for dinner."

"I'm all out of ideas for lunch."

"My breakfasts are monotonous."

"I'm in a rut."

Menu planning is an important responsibility for the homemaker. The health of her entire family depends largely on the meals she plans and prepares day after day. If you are one of the approximately thirty million American women who work outside of the home, you usually have to plan nutritious and appetizing menus for meals prepared (and often consumed) "on the run." Many other factors besides time for preparation enter into menu planning, such things as the size of the family, the age of its members, their likes and dislikes, income and budget, locality and occupation.

Someone in desperation wrote recently requesting an up-to-date book with menus for breakfast, lunch, and dinner for each of the three hundred and sixty-five days in the year. Such books are somewhat rare. While it seems that a year's menus would be an invaluable aid, they are not always practical. Good menus for a fisherman's family in Maine, would not fit an office worker's in southern California;

appropriate menus for a family of adults would not be suitable for a family with young children.

While all of these factors complicate the task, certain techniques and procedures make menu planning easier. Menu planning is both a science and an art.

The Science of Meal Planning

Here are some hints to help you plan effective menus. They can't change work to play, but they can make your chore more interesting and your meals less expensive.

- Have a set time for planning menus if possible, and think of each day as a unit rather than each meal separately.
- Plan menus in advance. Try a weekly or several-days-in-advance menu with an accompanying market list. This saves money and time by making marketing and meal preparation more efficient. The menu plan should be flexible enough to allow you to take advantage of good buys, use leftovers, and provide for unforeseen circumstances.
- Stay within your budget. The lower the allowance, the greater the challenge! You may save money by using foods in season, canning, drying, or freezing when seasonal foods are plentiful, and by preparing tasty dishes from leftovers. You can save time by doubling or tripling some recipes and freezing the extra for later use.
- Use the Daily Food Guide as the basis of menu planning. Adapt the Guide to each member of your family, from the toddler to grandparents. Include dishes the whole family enjoys. Your personal preferences should not dominate the menu planning; neither should food be avoided that one person dislikes.
- Establish a definite menu pattern. Here is a suggested basic menu pattern which translates the Daily Food Guide into three meals:

BREAKFAST	LUNCH OR SUPPER	DINNER
Fruit or juice or both	Protein dish	Protein dish
Cereal with milk or toast (or hot breads) or both	Fruit or vegetable	Vegetables
Egg or other protein	Bread, toast, or sandwich	Salad
Milk or other beverage	Margarine or butter	Bread or rolls
	Milk, hot or cold	Margarine or butter
		Hot or cold beverage

- To avoid monotony, change the pattern of a meal now and then. Plan it around the salad or soup or have a one-dish meal plus an interesting dessert.
- Serve a wide selection of food from meal to meal, vary your methods of preparation, and include foods of different texture at each meal. A rule sometimes suggested is to include at each meal something soft, something crisp and chewy, and something firm. To this could be added one food with satiety value.
- Serve heaviest meals in the morning and at noon if practical. Studies of both school children and adults of all ages show that greater mental and physical efficiency result all day if a fourth to a third of the daily nutrients are included at breakfast.

"It is the custom and order of society to take a slight breakfast. But this is not the best way to treat the stomach. At breakfast time the stomach is in a better condition to take care of more food than at the second or third meal of the day. The habit of eating a sparing breakfast and a large dinner is wrong. Make your breakfast correspond more nearly to the heartiest meal of the day."—Ellen G. White, *Counsels on Diet and Foods,* page 173.

- Plan the meals around the protein dish and distribute the protein, fat, and carbohydrate throughout the day, rather than concentrating it at one meal. Use sparingly foods such as sugar which contribute only "empty calories." Use fats moderately, largely avoiding fried or greasy foods.
- Maintain an up-to-date recipe file. Good recipes are both convenient and time-saving in planning menus. Be on the lookout for new recipes and cooking ideas in current periodicals, newspapers, and books. With ingenuity you can vary old recipes and develop new ones. International recipes will add zest to your menus. You may use family's favorite recipes often if you vary the other foods in the meal.
- Have special menus for occasions such as birthdays, anniversaries, holidays. Together with cookouts, patio meals, and picnics, they will add variety and spice to the usual routine.

The Art of Meal Planning

Meal planning is an art. Though not difficult, it requires thought and effort.

We eat with our eyes! Beautiful and colorful foods not only increase appetite but aid digestion. Clashing or drab colors are unpleasant. For example, what is more uninteresting and unappetizing than an all white meal?

An artistic meal includes foods in a variety of shapes and textures. Try visualizing a plate with round browned potatoes, a round scoop of cottage cheese, round tiny whole beets, and round little white onions. Even the texture is somewhat similar. Now substitute baked potatoes, sliced walnut loaf for the cottage cheese, and broccoli spears for the onions. Retain the beets. Shape and texture as well as color are improved.

Seasoning is an art and adds that "just right" touch. Herbs can add a subtle, delicate flavor to many recipes but watch it! Over seasoning can spoil the dish. Judicious use of strong and unusual flavors can be pleasing, but one such flavor at a meal is usually sufficient.

The aroma of a meal should be agreeable and tantalizing. The fragrance of fresh cut oranges or the whiff of baking bread, and many other savory odors, cause happy anticipation.

A garnish provides your distinctive, final touch. Nearly every food from soup to dessert may be garnished. The garnish should be appropriate, and it should harmonize with the food it adorns. It does not need to be elaborate. Simple garnishes are often the most effective and may be in better taste. Endless possibilities for garnishes can be found in magazines, restaurants, at friends' homes, and especially through use of your own ingenuity.

While foods are often improved in appearance by garnishing, meals may be artistic without added decoration simply because they have been planned with consideration for color, texture, shape, and flavor. The key to successful meal planning is simplicity, and the final touch to a pleasing meal is gracious service.

Menu Suggestions

These menus for breakfast, lunch, dinner, supper, and picnics follow the Daily Food Guide pattern. (Add margarine or butter to bread and vegetables; use milk and cream with hot beverages and cereals as desired.)

BREAKFASTS	LUNCHES OR SUPPERS	DINNERS
Orange juice Stewed prunes Seven-grain cereal Whole wheat toast Peanut butter Breakfast Cup	*Bean sandwich Raw apple Cocoa	*Royal salad Peas and carrots Mashed potatoes, gravy Oatmeal bread Berry pie Milk
Pineapple juice Fresh sliced peaches Shredded wheat Blueberry muffin Postum made with milk	Split pea soup Fresh strawberries 2 slices toast Milk or buttermilk	†Gluten Steaks Deluxe Corn on cob Green beans Sliced tomatoes Whole wheat bread Cupcake Milk
Mixed fruit juice Boysenberry toast with whipped cream Toasted cashew nuts Hot malted milk	†Brown rice with egg and curry sauce Fresh cherries Milk	†Soy cheese patties Baked banana squash Buttered asparagus tips Tossed green salad Rye bread Orange cake Buttermilk
½ grapefruit Ruskets with dates Cornbread Honey Cocoa	Cream of tomato soup, with crackers Cottage cheese and pineapple salad 2 slices pumpernickel bread	†Mushroom nutmeat potpie Baked yams Spinach, lemon Avocado salad Rolls Apple strudel Milk

---

*See chapter 5, page 44 for recipes.

†Recipes for these dishes can be found in the companion cookbook series to this volume, *Vegetarian Cookery*.

BREAKFASTS	**LUNCHES OR SUPPERS**	**DINNERS**
Sliced orange Baked apple Milk toast Poached egg Cereal coffee	Fresh fruit compote †Nut butter and diced cucumber sandwich Ovaltine	†Soyameat casserole Green peas Mashed turnips †Grated carrot and coconut salad Whole wheat bread Molasses cookies Milk
Cantaloupe Canned pears Oatmeal and raisins Creamed nutmeat on zweibach Postum	†Cream of potato soup with parsley flakes Orange slices and cream cheese Coconut sticks Buttermilk	†Spaghetti Marzetti Tossed green salad Toasted garlic bread Angel cake and sherbet Milk
Tomato juice Apricot sauce Scrambled egg Rye toast Breakfast cup	Fresh fruit salad Glutenburger on buns Hot malted milk	†Spanish lentils Baked russet potatoes Mixed greens, lemon Coleslaw Cornbread Pecan pie Milk

Picnic Lunches

1)

Potato salad
Baked great northern beans
Sliced tomatoes and lettuce
Olives
Cloverleaf rolls
†Date chews
Iced punch or hot drink

2)

Baked noodles lasagne or garbanzos with dumplings
Tossed salad
Relishes (olives, radishes, celery, cucumbers)
Garlic bread or French rolls
Cantaloupe a la mode
Iced punch or hot drink

Housecleaning or Washday Dinners

1)

Split pea soup
Tossed vegetable salad
Garlic rye toast
Milk

2)

Baked beans
Salad—vegetable or fruit with cottage cheese
Brown bread
Milk

Cookout

Roasted corn on cob
Sliced tomatoes and cucumbers
Roasted vegetable weiners in rolls
Watermelon
Hot cocoa

---

†Recipes for these dishes can be found in the companion cookbook series to this volume, *Vegetarian Cookery*.

Good Nutrition on a Budget

"Housewives Are Grumbling" bannered the headline in a news weekly; and no wonder—food prices were rising. Many American families spend more for food than for any other item budgeted.

Even with rising food costs, however, you can reduce the amount you spend for food and at the same time improve the nutritive quality of the meals you serve. How do you accomplish this neat little trick? Not by sleight of hand, but by wise planning and careful buying.

The amount you spend for food should, of course, be geared to your family's needs. The food items purchased and amount spent vary according to the total income of the family, its size, and the ages, sex, activity, occupation, and health of its members. Climate, locality, marketing facilities, and personal preferences also influence the food budget.

On average incomes one fifth to one third, and on very low incomes one half or more, may need to be budgeted for food. The lower the income the more difficult your task of providing nutritious and appealing meals, but saving on food costs does not have to mean serving less food or food of inferior quality.

With each addition to the family, the food costs increase; but the proportionate cost per person becomes less. The NRC Daily Recommended Allowances on pages 16, 17 shows the differences that age and sex make in nutritional requirements. Infants and small children require food that is different from and perhaps more expensive than that for other members of the family. Children need more food as they grow older. Moderately active boys and men require more calories than moderately active girls and women. During pregnancy and lactation nutritional needs are greater. The elderly need nourishing, attractive, easily digested foods to appeal to their diminishing appetites. Persons in poor health may require special diets. The more active the person, or the colder his climate, the more calories he needs. This does not mean that his food costs must increase, because many high calorie foods are low in cost.

Where you live and the activities you enjoy may affect your food budget. For example, living costs are often higher in cities than in rural areas, although not always. Eating meals out and frequent entertaining can make your food costs soar. If you have only a limited amount to spend for food, your family may have to curtail some of these pleasures. Home gardens and canning, freezing and preserving at the peak of the season, are usually good practices financially.

Today, buying food for the home is "big business" and a real challenge. More than 8,000 different items confront you on supermarket shelves—five times the amount of twenty years ago, and increasing daily! An estimated thirty to forty new items are added every month. No wonder shoppers often feel bewildered.

The thrifty shopper considers the amount of time and energy she can spend in shopping and food preparation. Modern homemakers are said to spend considerably more time shopping than their mothers did, but less time cooking. If you are employed outside the home, convenience foods may be a necessity even though the "extra built-in service" costs more.

If you plan your menus in advance, you can check them against supplies on hand, and then make out your market list. In this way you can make the best purchases in the shortest time, avoid haphazard shopping, and plan a more even distribution of expensive items.

With the shopping list in hand, the next consideration is how to get the most for your money in each food group. Choose as wide a variety of foods as your budget allows.

To buy wisely, compare prices and yields and read labels before purchasing. Information such as the drained weight, size or count, and contents can help you make a wise and economical choice of canned goods. The ingredients are listed in the descending order of the amounts included—the main ingredient first. Canned whole fruits and vegetables cost more than slices, chunks, or halves.

Note brand names, but remember that those less highly advertised may be more economical and of equally good quality. But one pitfall to watch for is the cheaper brands that sometimes contain less solids. To avoid buying such items, check the drained weight and the serving yields. In some instances a well-known brand may cost a few cents more initially but yield an extra serving and actually be more economical. If the drained weight is not given on the label, try shaking the can lightly to determine the amount of liquid to solids. A choice grade sometimes serves the purpose as well as a fancy grade and at a considerable saving. This is the case when a recipe does not specify a large size or uniform size and shape.

To aid homemakers in planning and spending effectively, the United States Department of Agriculture has furnished tables showing the foods that yield the most nutritive value for each dollar spent. These tables (see pages 33-35) are based on 1961 food prices but reflect, in general, adequate comparison for today.

Purchasing the Cereal and Bread Group. The cereal and bread group are the least expensive and, next to fats and oils, the most concentrated sources of energy. They are an inexpensive source of protein, thiamine, riboflavin, and iron, as well as other nutrients.

Whole grain breads and cereals are the best investment with enriched or restored products a close second. The kind of bread or cereal affects the cost. Dry cereals may cost three times as much as cooked cereals. The popped, puffed, and sugar-coated ones give the least value for the money spent. Bread is less expensive than rolls, and purchasing day-old bread at a bakery or distributor's outlet cuts costs.

Buying the Milk Group Is Good Economy. Foods in the milk group sometimes seem expensive, but they supply so many important nutrients that it is false economy to use less than the amounts recommended in the Daily Food Guide.

Milk, whether whole, evaporated, non-fat, or buttermilk, contains protein of high quality and is the cheapest source of calcium and riboflavin. The price of whole versus canned or dry milk varies considerably. For example, reconstituted powdered non-fat milk usually costs one third or less and evaporated milk two thirds the price of whole fresh milk.

A good economy measure is to combine whole milk with an equal

Chart 1.—CALORIE YIELD For One Dollar Spent

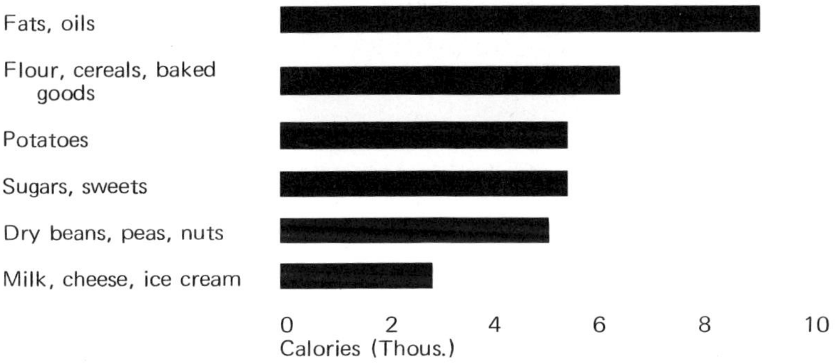

Chart 2.—PROTEIN YIELD For One Dollar Spent

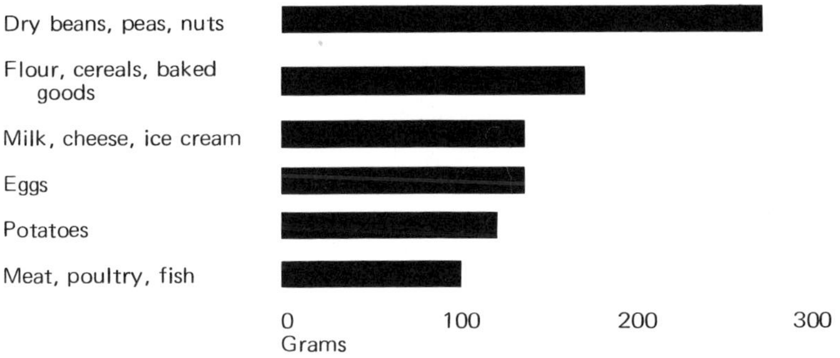

Chart 3.—CALCIUM YIELD For One Dollar Spent

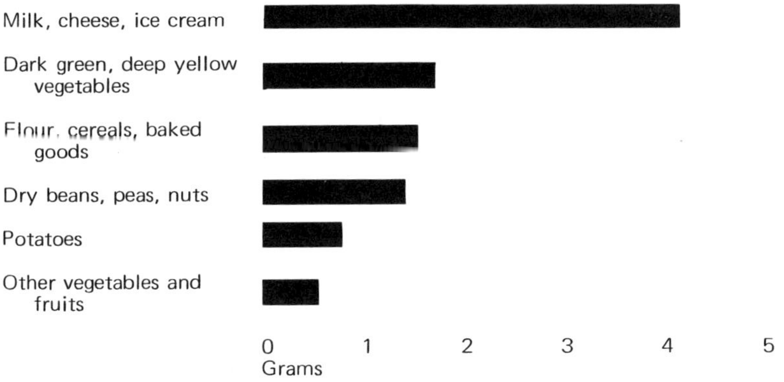

Chart 4.—IRON YIELD For One Dollar Spent

Chart 5.—VITAMIN A YIELD For One Dollar Spent

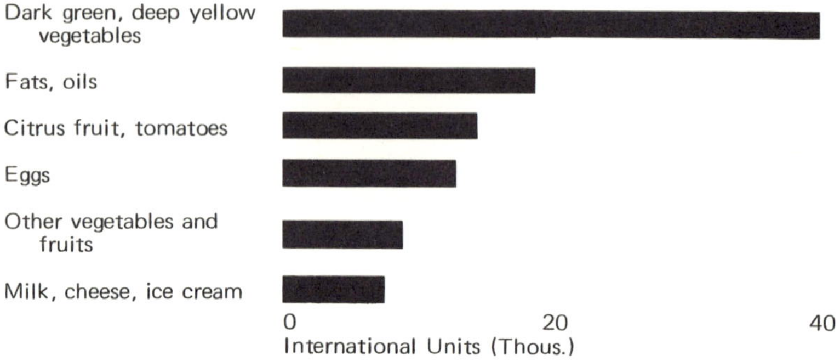

Chart 6.—THIAMINE YIELD For One Dollar Spent

Chart 7.—RIBOFLAVIN YIELD For One Dollar Spent

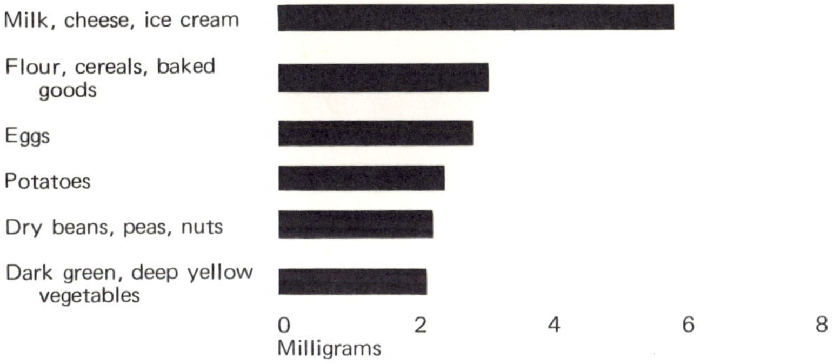

Chart 8.—NIACIN YIELD For One Dollar Spent

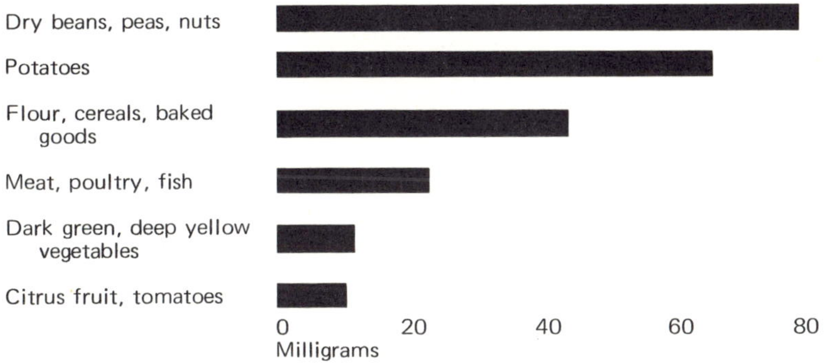

Chart 9.—ASCORBIC ACID YIELD For One Dollar Spent

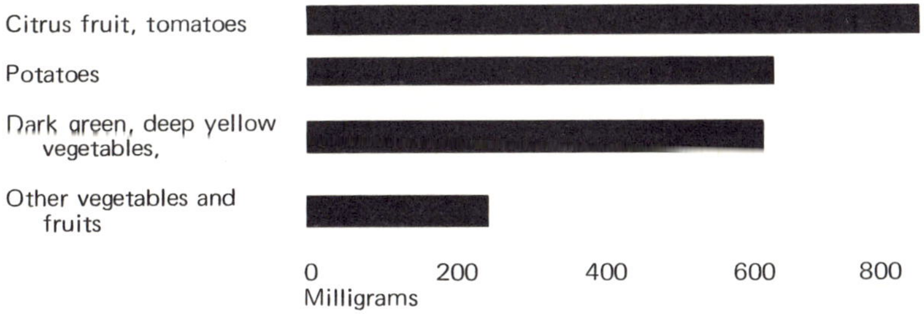

amount of reconstituted non-fat milk. Some people use non-fat milk almost exclusively because of its lower cholesterol content. If you can store it in air tight containers and keep it in a cool, dry place, you can make a considerable saving by purchasing dry non-fat milk in bulk. It is safest to choose a pasteurized variety.

Using Economical Protein Foods. Vegetable protein sources are economical in price, but as a whole they are not as high quality as the animal proteins—milk, cheese, eggs (and flesh foods). Milk used as recommended in the Daily Food Guide will supplement the protein value of vegetable foods, and these inexpensive foods may be relied upon with confidence as a protein source. Research demonstrates that many vegetable proteins complement one another to produce high quality protein; but until more is known about supplementary values, it is wise to include milk and eggs in the diet of growing children and teen-agers, especially during times of stress such as illness; and in women during pregnancy and lactation. Another important reason for the inclusion of some foods of animal origin is that vegetable foods do not appear to provide adequate vitamin B_{12}.

With this in mind check charts 1 through 9 (see pages 33-35) and note that peanuts and dry beans, peas, lentils, and garbanzos are not only an economical source of protein but also furnish more iron and niacin for your dollar than any other food. There are a variety of dried legumes. In fact a different kind of legume could be used in some form every day for several weeks without repetition. Dishes prepared from legumes, nuts, eggs, cheese, and processed vegetable protein can be highly nutritious at a very reasonable cost. For example, a patty made with nuts, cereal, and cottage cheese yields about ten grams of high quality protein at a cost of only about five cents.

Cottage cheese is an economical source of high quality protein—one-half cup will furnish about one-fourth (15 grams) of the day's protein requirement for an adult. One ounce of cheddar cheese costs about the same but contributes only half the amount of protein. Cheddar does furnish slightly more calcium than cottage cheese, however.

Eggs vie with milk as a good source of protein and riboflavin. They also contribute other minerals and vitamins such as iron and vitamin A. To economize, you may extend eggs by using them in patties, loaves, and creamed dishes.

Only high-quality, clean eggs should be purchased. They should be refrigerated at the market and should be stored immediately in your home refrigerator. It is poor economy to purchase cracked or dirty eggs as salmonella infection is readily spread in this way. The use of raw eggs is questionable. Only by thoroughly cooking eggs, it appears, can the salmonella and other harmful organisms in them be destroyed.

Paying more for white (or brown) eggs is not good economy. The shell color has nothing to do with the nutritive value, grade, flavor, or cooking performance of the egg. Grade AA (or A) eggs are preferred for poaching. Grade B eggs may be used at considerable saving in cooking and baking when appearance is not important. Considering the size (small, medium, or large) the United States Department of Agriculture states, "If there is less than a seven-cent price spread per dozen between one size and the next smaller size in the same grade, you will get more for your money by buying the larger size."

Stretching the Vegetable and Fruit Dollar. Fruits and vegetables, if purchased in season, are among the most economical items on the menu. They add nutrients, variety, and color.

Select fruits and vegetables that are crisp, firm, and plump. Most fruits should be neither hard nor soft. Wilt, bruises, or decay spots usually indicate poor quality and should be avoided. Fruits and vegetables of irregular size or with blemishes which do not affect the quality are frequently good buys. Root vegetables should be smooth, firm, and clean. Beets and turnips with fresh tops provide extra value as you can use the tops for greens.

Dark green leafy and deep yellow vegetables are by far the most economical source of vitamin A (carotene) and are second only to milk as an inexpensive source of calcium (about one third to one half that of milk). Leafy vegetables are a good source of iron.

When it comes to ascorbic acid, citrus fruits and tomatoes usually rate as your best buys. The purchase price varies with the season and the supply. As with all perishables, they demand proper storing and preparation in order to realize the best economy.

According to the tables, the value received for dollar spent is somewhat impressive for potatoes. Because they have been labeled high in calories, many people avoid them; but they are nevertheless a good food—an economical source of thiamine, iron, ascorbic acid, and niacin, and a fairly economical source of protein and calcium.

In summary, here are some ideas to help you save dollars in your food budget:

Dollar Savers

- Plan menus well in advance (three to four days or a week). Make your plans flexible enough to allow for unexpected guests, good food buys, and use of leftovers.
- To save time and expensive impulse buying, make a list, putting like items together.
- Take advantage of good buys. Check newspapers and market ads for specials.
- Compare relative costs of foods when fresh, canned, frozen, dried, et cetera, and estimate the cost per pound, ounce, or serving of each.
- Buy staples in quantity or in large-sized containers if you have ample storage and if the food can be used to good advantage without waste. Bulk items usually cost less.
- Limit purchases of perishable items to amounts that can be used while in top-quality condition.
- Become well acquainted with varieties of fresh fruits and vegetables, their characteristics, and seasons, so that wise choices can be made.
- Buy foods in season, produced locally, and when in plentiful supply. Food costs less and is best at the peak of the season. This is also the best time for canning, preserving, and freezing.
- Extend expensive protein foods by mixing with less expensive items.
- Buy prepared foods such as TV dinners only when necessary to save time or if less expensive than home prepared. Check quality against price.
- Be a label reader.
- Be alert to "hidden costs."
- Avoid waste from poor cooking habits by:
  - Utilizing leftovers.
  - Paring carefully and thinly and saving ends of asparagus, celery tops, vegetable peelings to use in stew or in stock for soup or gravy.
  - Using liquid from cooked vegetables.
  - Avoiding scorching and overcooking.
  - Scraping kettles thoroughly.
- You have the well-being of your family in your hands—choose to purchase health rather than sickness by wise buying practices.

Meals That Travel: Lunches

Millions of men, women, and children eat from lunch boxes every day. If you are a lunch packer, you know that making good meals that travel is a constant challenge. It takes care, ingenuity, and imagination to make them as inviting and nourishing as other meals.

Throughout the United States the National School Lunch Program serves type "A" lunches which conform to standards set by the Department of Agriculture. We can adapt these to the home-prepared lunch. They are: (1) Make it well-balanced; (2) Make it attractive; (3) Make it taste good; and (4) Make it generous.

Make It Well-balanced. The wise lunch packer who is, preferably, someone other than the eater, will make use of the Daily Food Guide in planning lunches. Whether the lunch goes to school, work, or picnic, the same principles apply as for the meal that is eaten at home. A nutritious lunch should furnish one fourth to one third of the daily requirement of nutrients.

Fit the lunch into your daily and weekly menu pattern. Adjust for age and activity needs of the lunch carrier. An outdoor worker may need twice as many calories as an office worker. A large active boy will need more than a moderately active girl. Teen-age girls tend to be "fussy" and prefer dainty, attractive food; and they frequently diet to reduce. Some teen age boys, on the other hand, seem chronically hungry. Climate also should influence the size and types of lunches. When the weather is cold, lunches need to be larger and of heavier quality and should contain some hot foods.

Suggested foods to be included in the type "A" home lunch apply also to the carried lunch: one serving of protein such as cottage cheese, egg, or legumes (this may be the sandwich filling); one cup or more of milk, hot or cold, or in soup; three fourths cup or more of vegetable or fruit; one slice or more of whole grain or enriched bread. A good nutritious sandwich can be the backbone of the lunch. Slices of bread can sometimes be replaced with buns or rolls.

Change the meal pattern occasionally using a hearty salad, soup, or hot dish in place of the usual sandwich. Raw, toasted, or salted mixed nuts add variety to your meal, or they may be chopped in sandwich spreads. Make use of natural sweets such as dates and dried fruits for dessert. A good rule is, "No calories without minerals and vitamins."

Make It Look Attractive. Eye appeal does much to determine the zest with which a lunch is eaten. Here are a few suggestions for preparing attractive lunches:

1. Pack carefully and with order.
   Heavier things should go on the bottom.
   Napkins, at least two, should be neatly folded on top. Sometimes colored, flower, or picture napkins can be substituted for the white.
   Sandwiches stay fresher if neatly wrapped. You might try cutting them in different shapes for variety. Make the filling moist but not runny, and spread filling to edge of bread.
2. Use attractive containers, sized to fit individual needs. For small children you might use—
   Colored plastic boxes or cups.
   Small jars with painted designs or colorful stickers on lid or side.
3. Choose good quality fruits and vegetables.
4. Tempt with pleasing color and texture, such as:
   shiny red apples, peaches, big oranges, cherry tomatoes, crisp lettuce, cabbage wedges, olives, et cetera.
5. Provide color contrast by using, for example, a fresh or maraschino cherry with stem to garnish a fruit compote, or a teaspoon of red or green jelly or a sprig of mint. Poke carrot and celery sticks through pitted black olives.

Make It Taste Good. A lunch may be nutritious and beautiful, but if it is to be enjoyed and eaten with relish it must also taste good.

It should be fresh and nicely seasoned; hot foods should be kept hot and cold foods kept cold in a thermos.

Make the lunch one you would enjoy, keeping in mind the particular tastes of the lunch carrier. If possible, include a favorite item or something different every day. Add something fresh and crisp and crunchy to chew and something like milk, juice, or hot soup or beverage to drink. Different breads and fillings in the sandwiches add interesting variety.

Something tart whets the appetite and is good if the lunch is otherwise bland. Care should be taken to avoid placing foods with strong odors in the packed lunch box. Avoid, too, repeating in the lunch the same food served at the other meals of the day.

Make It Generous. Consider the individual for whom you are packing the lunch. Does he (or she) like to eat well? Then pack ample food. Or does he have a finicky appetite? In this case avoid including so much as to discourage him from eating. Consider the length of the lunch period. If it is only twenty minutes, plan a lunch that can be eaten comfortably in that time. For example, a thermos of soup is nourishing and can be drunk quickly. Oranges peeled and sectioned and apples quartered and wrapped in plastic are also convenient to eat and nutritious and look tempting enough to attract even the child who tends to slight lunch for play. If your child is one of these, make his meal concentrated and easy to eat.

Time Savers for the Lunch Packer

If you have several lunches to pack every day and if you have space enough in your kitchen, set aside a "Packer's Corner" for work space and a particular drawer, shelf, or even cupboard for storing equipment and supplies. Outlaw all other activities from your corner. To stock your supply drawer (or shelf or cupboard) you will need such items as lunch boxes and thermoses, foil, waxed paper, plastic wrap, paper napkins, plastic containers, and disposable forks, spoons, and cups. In addition, you may also want to reserve especially for your packing area such frequently used materials as sharp knives, spoons and forks, measuring cups, a spatula, a cutting board, straws, miniature salt shakers, and such edible staples as bread, salad dressing, nuts, peanut butter, et cetera.

Plan ahead. Think lunches when planning the weekly menus,

when shopping, and when cooking. To avoid the last minute rush in the morning, do everything you possibly can the night before. Prepare and refrigerate sandwich fillings; wash and wrap lettuce, watercress, and other vegetables; wash and shine apples; place nuts, cookies, or dried fruits in bags; boil and shell eggs; cream the butter or keep at the right temperature for spreading. It's a good idea to refrigerate the thermos the night before for cold beverages.

The "Somethings" That Make Lunch "Something"

Variety of Bread

You can choose from an amazing variety of different types of bread:

Corn
French
Graham
Herb
Oatmeal
Potato
Pumpernickel
Rye
Soy
Seven-grain
White
Whole wheat

Fruit bread:
- Apricot nut
- Banana
- Date nut
- Raisin
- Raisin nut
- Orange
- Boston brown

Rolls:
- Butter flake
- Cloverleaf
- Parker House
- Sandwich buns
- Wiener rolls

Bread sticks:
- Corn
- Coconut
- Whole wheat
- Walnut

Crackers
Croutons
Muffins
Zwiebach

Variety in Butter Spreads

The following items may be mixed individually with butter or in various combinations:

Savorex, Sovex, or Vegex.
Clipped parsley and onion or garlic.
Chopped parsley and lemon juice.
Cucumber, finely chopped, with lemon juice and salt.
Chopped, sautéd mushrooms with lemon juice.
Minced herbs.
Crushed, toasted sesame seeds.
Chopped nuts.
Honey.

Variety in Sandwich Fillings

Hard-boiled eggs, chopped or mashed, with mayonnaise and:
- Chopped olives.
- Cottage cheese.
- Mashed avocado.
- Mashed or pureed garbanzos, chopped celery, onion, and lemon juice.
- Chopped celery.
- Savita, Sovex, Savorex, Marmite, or Vegex.

Eggs, scrambled with:
- Savorex, onions, and sour cream.
- Diced tomatoes, celery, and onions.
- Cottage cheese.
- Mashed garbanzos, Savorex, onions, mayonnaise.

Cream or neufchâtel cheese is delicious plain or mixed with:
- Savorex (and spread on rye or herb breads).
- Softened with milk (fruit bread).
- Chopped nuts.
- Chopped olives, black, green, stuffed, or green ripe.

Chopped dates, dried fruits, or pineapple.
- Chopped celery, green onion or chives, radishes, cucumbers, bell peppers, or other vegetables or vegetable combinations.
- Jams, jellies, marmalade, cranberry relish, apple butter, or apricot puree.
- (Cottage cheese may be substituted for the cream or neufchâtel cheese, if pressed through a sieve.)

Dried fruit, chopped or ground with nuts, lemon juice, and honey.

Peanut butter, plain or emulsified with water, and mixed with these:
- Crushed pineapple, mashed bananas, and chopped dates or raisins.
- Sliced tomatoes, finely grated carrots, chopped celery, and radishes or cucumbers.
- Honey, jelly, jam, marmalade, apple butter, or cranberry relish.

Beans or other legumes may be mashed and mixed with:
- Celery, onion, tomato, bell pepper, or combinations of these.

Nutmeat, light or dark, diced or mashed, with:
- Celery, tomatoes, onion, and mayonnaise.
- Chopped olives and mayonnaise.

Vegetables make good fillings, such as:

Sliced radishes or cucumbers with sour cream.

Grated carrot and celery with nuts or coconut.

Tomato and lettuce, plain or with avocado.

Avocado with lemon and salt or mayonnaise.

Glutenburger patties in buns with relishes.

Vegetarian wieners in long buns with relishes.

Sliced cold loaf or patties of gluten, nutmeat, soyameat, cottage cheese.

Soyameat, plain, or chopped and mixed with mayonnaise, celery, onion, and Tartex.

Welcome Surprises

A rosebud or other flower packed with lunch.

A love note from Mother.

A small box of raisins.

A cup cake or cookies with decorative frosting.

Dried fruit rolled in nuts or coconut.

Recipe Suggestions

Stuff prunes (or dates or figs) with:

Mashed banana and peanut butter.

Cream cheese thinned with orange juice and with grated rind.

Stuff celery sticks with:

Cream cheese or cottage cheese and pimiento.

Pig-in-a-blanket:

Cut crusts from thinly sliced fresh bread, spread with butter or salad dressing, and roll the bread around an asparagus spear and sprig of watercress or a small vegetarian wiener. Hold together with toothpick.

Stuffed tomatoes:

Cream cheese or cottage cheese with chives or with finely chopped celery, radishes, green onion, and parsley. Sliced and scored cucumbers (unpeeled) make a nice garnish.

Royal salad:

Dice equal parts of nutmeat (browned in oven), celery, and hard cooked eggs and mix with a generous amount of mayonnaise. Garnish with a little grated hard-boiled egg yolk or tomato wedges. (If diced finely, this salad may be used as a hearty sandwich filling.)

Neapolitan Salad:
Add peas to the above salad.

Fruit cup—juicy combinations of fruit, fresh and canned, make good eating with most lunches. Combining any two or three of the following is delicious: Apricots, peaches, pears, pineapple, berries, cherries, and oranges. Bananas, if desired, may be added just before completing the lunch. Coconut with orange or pineapple is also appetizing.

Menu Suggestions for the Meal That Travels

Cold	*Hot*
†Gluten steaks deluxe sandwich Tomato, carrot and celery sticks Milk Dates stuffed with nuts	†Washington chowder Whole wheat bread with Savorex butter sandwich Jellied fruit and cottage cheese salad Cupcake
Deviled egg Lettuce and tomato sandwich Milk Apple and peanuts	Navy beans Boston brown bread Stuffed celery Milk Sectioned orange
Garbanzo sandwich Olives Fruit salad Milk Oatmeal cookie	†Spaghetti Marzetti Relishes (celery, olives, radishes) Milk Pear
*Grated carrot sandwich *Royal salad Milk Grapes	Cream of lentil soup Zwieback and butter Orange coconut cup Cookie Nuts

*See recipes or serving suggestions, pages 142, 143.

† Recipes for these dishes can be found in the companion cookbook series to this volume, *Vegetarian Cookery*.

Potato and egg salad
Tomato and lettuce
Milk
Whole wheat rolls and butter
Peach

Glutenburger in bun
Fruit compote
Milk
Nut cookie

Hot chocolate
Vegetarian wieners in finger rolls
Jellied fruit mold
Date and nut squares

Protein Facts

Proteins resemble a jigsaw puzzle in which each of the pieces—the amino acids—join together to form the complete protein molecule. And, like a jigsaw puzzle, if just one piece is missing, the design is incomplete.

There are about twenty amino acids. Each one is made of carbon, oxygen, and hydrogen, with the added bonus of nitrogen which makes protein different from the carbohydrates and fat. Like the twenty-six letters of the alphabet, which can be combined to form many different words of numerous letters, the amino acids can be combined in specific sequences to form protein molecules containing thousands of amino acids.

Gerardus Johannes Mulder, a Dutch physician and chemist, described protein as "unquestionably the most important of all known substances in the organic kingdom. Without it no life appears possible on our planet." The name protein comes from a Greek word meaning "to take first place."

And protein still takes first place, nutritionwise. Supplying adequate protein to the people, especially the children, of the world is the major nutritional problem today and is of international concern. Efforts to find a solution involve not only nutritionists, biochemists, and food technologists but statesmen also.

But protein is needed not only in faraway lands; it is essential to you and your family, your health and vitality. Since all living substances contain protein, it is necessary for life—your life. Why is protein so important? What does it do in the body and for the body?

It is a protein—hemoglobin in the red blood cells—which carries oxygen from the lungs to the tissues and carbon dioxide from the tissues to the lungs. It is proteins—albumin and globulins—which are involved in the exchange of water and minerals between the blood, lymph, and tissues. If the protein level in the serum decreases, the fluid balance becomes upset, water accumulates, and edema results.

It is proteins—enzymes and most hormones—which affect metabolism. It is proteins—gamma globulins—which as antibodies can destroy bacteria, viruses, and other microorganisms in the body and sometimes confer temporary or permanent immunity to specific diseases. Proteins also serve as buffers in the complex system which keeps the blood in a slightly alkaline condition.

Much of our knowledge about protein and its functions comes from research in this century. To grow, a child needs ample protein, and the need does not stop when he grows from youth to adulthood. Throughout life the proteins in all living tissues are continually broken down and built up. Because of this the daily diet should supply adequate amounts of protein even after the growing years are over.

One gram of protein furnishes four calories, so some of your energy may come from protein. Since your body's need for energy must be met, proteins will be used if carbohydrates and fats are low in the diet. Carbohydrates are sometimes called protein sparers because they supply fuel and energy and spare protein for its other important functions.

Plants are able with the help of the sun to make their own protein from carbon dioxide, water, and the nitrogen in the air and soil; but human beings and animals must get their protein from plants or from other animals. The proteins of each plant and animal species differ from every other. Proteins in oats or rye, for example, are not the same as those of wheat. Even the proteins in various parts of the body differ—muscle, skin, and hemoglobin proteins are not the same.

Each protein is a large and complex puzzle, usually containing thousands of amino acids joined in a specific sequence. If this sequence is broken by one amino acid missing or out of place, the results may be serious. For example, in the cases of persons suffering from sickle-cell anemia (when a specific amino acid is replaced by a different one) the life span is shortened.

To be absorbed from the digestive tract, protein has to be broken down by digestive enzymes into the original amino acids. If a large molecule of protein were to be taken directly into the blood without being broken down into amino acids, allergic reactions would occur. Thus complete proteins replenish the body's amino acid pool. The muscles contain one third of your total body protein, the skin contains one fifth, and various other parts of your body contain the remainder of your total proteins.

The terms "essential" and "nonessential" are sometimes used to characterize amino acids. Your body can synthesize some amino acids but others it cannot. Those which cannot be synthesized are called essential amino acids and must be present in the food. They are leucine, isoleucine, lysine, methionine, phenylalanine, threonine, tryptophane, valine (and also histidine for children). The so-called nonessential amino acids can be manufactured by your body from other nutrients or from the essential amino acids.

Probably you have heard about complete, partially complete, and incomplete proteins. Such terms refer to the amount and proportion of essential amino acids present in a protein. Complete proteins have all the essential amino acids in sufficient amounts and proportions to support growth and maintain life, even when they are the only protein in the diet.

Partially complete proteins have all of the essential amino acids but in inadequate amounts or incorrect proportions. When they are the only protein in the diet they will sustain life but not growth. Incomplete proteins lack one or more of the essential amino acids and will neither support growth nor maintain life.

It is seldom that only one protein is used in a meal; therefore the classification of complete or incomplete usually affects only those individuals with limited food available or those on dietaries used for experimentation.

Foods from animal sources such as milk, cheese, eggs, meat, fish, and poultry contain complete proteins and thus supply all of the essential amino acids. Soybean, garbanzo, and peanut proteins have been compared with animal protein in quality. Green leafy vegetables also furnish excellent protein but in such minute amounts that they do not contribute much to the protein requirements.

Proteins in grains, nuts, most legumes, vegetables, and fruits are frequently classified as partially complete. Fortunately proteins of different foods can supplement each other. A meal which combines two or more foods with partially complete or incomplete proteins may provide protein of good quality which will support life and promote growth.

Good amino acid balance can be obtained by combining cereals with legumes, nuts, milk, cheese, or eggs. Throughout the ages people have practiced supplementation of protein instinctively. In the United States, for instance, a typical breakfast contains cereal and milk.

Primitive societies have combined grains and legumes in their diets for centuries, but the value of the supplementation is just now being realized. Many cereal proteins are low in the amino acid lysine, but fairly well-supplied with sulphur-containing amido acids. Legumes, on the other hand, are good sources of lysine but low in sulphur-containing amino acids. Thus legumes and cereals may supplement each other. One study found that a combination of beans and rice resulted in a nutritive value similar to that of a complete protein. Some legumes and nuts may supplement each other and are good sources of minerals and vitamins as well. (See chart pages 33-35.)

Digestibility of a protein bears on its nutritive value. Your cooking methods also affect the value you receive from the proteins in your food. Some of the amino acids, such as lysine, are unstable and may be destroyed by overheating, toasting, or frying. However, cooking in water improves the digestibility of beans and wheat proteins.

Since every protein contains nitrogen, the protein needs of people and animals have been investigated by nitrogen balance studies. These studies are customarily carried on for a number of days or weeks in order to determine the variations from day to day. There are two considerations in nitrogen balance studies: first, the intake of protein in the food; and, second, the output of nitrogen in the body excretions. The intake of protein is determined by chemical analysis of the foods or by calculating from tables of nutritive values. The output of nitrogen is ascertained by laboratory tests.

When the nitrogen in the food is more than the amount excreted by the body, you are in positive nitrogen balance. When the intake equals the excretion, there is nitrogen equilibrium. In contrast, if the nitrogen intake is less than the output you are in negative nitrogen balance.

A normal adult should be in nitrogen equilibrium. During growth, pregnancy, and lactation, the need for protein is increased. New tissues are being built and nitrogen is retained. In other words, there should be positive nitrogen balance.

In wasting diseases, burns, starvation, and fevers, there is much tissue breakdown. If the supply of protein in the diet is low at such times the body will draw from its own tissues to supply the lack and there will be a negative nitrogen balance.

Protein Sources. Protein of good quality can be obtained from both animal and plant sources.

Milk and milk products, eggs, meat, poultry, and fish are protein foods of animal origin.

Plant proteins are contained in legumes (beans, peas, lentils, garbanzos, and peanuts), nuts (such as walnuts, pecans, cashews, almonds), and cereals (wheat, rye, oats, corn, rice, barley, millet). Vegetables and fruits contribute only a small portion of protein. Seeds of sesame, cotton, sunflower, pumpkin, and squash have a relatively high percentage of protein.

Some spun soybean products and vegetable protein foods manufactured from legumes, nuts, cereals, wheat gluten, and soybeans approach the taste and texture of meat. Available in canned or, in the case of several, frozen form, these products make inexpensive main dishes which are both nutritious and tasty. Food stores such as supermarkets and health food stores carry them in most areas of the United States.

Plant protein sources, if properly chosen and combined, can meet the needs for the essential amino acids and contribute to an adequate diet.

Protein Requirement. Karl von Voit, a German physiologist and nutritionist, established the first protein requirements in 1881. He believed that people needed 118 grams of protein daily to sustain good nutrition. He based his conclusions on surveys of German workers in Berlin.

Later at Yale University, Russell H. Chittenden, who was the first physiological chemistry teacher in America, questioned von Voit's standards. He experimented on himself and others, including young athletes, during periods of six months to more than a year and found that diets containing only 53 grams of protein a day could maintain proper balance.

In 1920 Henry C. Sherman of Columbia University analyzed all of the available evidence on protein requirements. He came to the conclusion that one half gram of protein daily per kilogram (2.2 pounds equals one kilogram) of body weight was sufficient to meet the body's needs. Further experiments have shown that even less protein is sufficient if the protein quality is good. Dr. Sherman, however, advised a fifty percent mark-up from the one half gram as a "margin of safety."

The National Research Council Recommended Daily Dietary Allowances provide a safety margin and suggest 0.9 grams per kilogram of body weight. This means 65 grams of protein each day for a normal healthy adult man weighing about 154 pounds (70 kilograms) and 55 grams each day for a woman weighing 128 pounds (58 kilograms). During pregnancy 65 grams are recommended and 75 during lactation. The amounts for children vary with size and age.

Protein Deficiency. A news picture, showing a pitiful group of pot-bellied, spindly-legged children with sad, drawn faces, flashed onto the television screen. It came from a faraway country, but it could have been taken in Egypt, Mexico, India, Central America, Brazil, Southeast Asia, the West Indies, or certain areas of the United States. Those children and millions more suffer from protein deficiency.

In areas where dietary protein is poor in quality or scarce, malnutrition especially during infancy and childhood is common. Protein deficiency is particularly prevalent in the low socio-economic brackets among infants and children, pregnant and nursing women, and elderly people.

Malnutrition may occur, even in America, when there is a low protein intake due to lack of knowledge or misinformation regarding protein needs; when fasting or dieting without medical advice; or when excessive loss of protein takes place as with hemorrhage, burns, fevers, wounds, and starvation.

Kwashiorkor, a widespread pronounced form of malnutrition, results largely from protein deficiency. The condition is known as *shibi gachaki* in Japan, *mehlnahrshaden* in Germany, *male de farina* in Italy, and *sindrome pluricarencial infantil* in Central America. Economic, social, sanitary, and educational factors contribute to its high incidence.

It occurs most often in infants after weaning, when the diet which replaces the mother's milk is very deficient in protein and consists largely of carbohydrates. Among the symptoms are malnutrition, edema, lesions of the skin resembling pellagra, apathy, loss of appetite, diarrhea, poor resistance to infection, retarded growth, and discoloration of the hair.

The treatment of kwashiorkor includes administering protein of high nutritive value. When reconstituted non-fat milk was fed to a group of children with kwashiorkor, they made dramatic improvement. A good diet with all the essential nutrients from available local food is given as soon as tolerated. Supplementation of the diet in the weaning and postweaning periods contributes most to preventing kwashiorkor. Vegetable protein mixtures have been used satisfactorily in place of milk in Central America, the Congo, India, South Africa, and Lebanon. As an example, a vegetable preparation called Incaparina has been used successfully in Central America.

Vegetable proteins are being studied in the laboratories of many countries in their efforts to find a solution to the world's protein problem.

The Calorie Counters: Carbohydrates and Fats

"How many calories in this pie?"

"How many calories in a milkshake?"

Do you ever ask these questions? Most people associate calories with weight gain or loss and want to learn to count calories. Some also inquire, "What is a calorie?"

Actually a calorie is a measure of energy, or heat. Bodies are living machines that require fuel to keep going. The large calorie used in nutrition is the kilo calorie or kcal and has been defined as the amount of heat required to raise one kilogram of water one degree Centigrade (or four pounds of water one degree Fahrenheit); but the definition means little to most of us unless it is associated with food substances.

What are the calorie counters? Carbohydrates, fats, and proteins all supply calories. Protein is not a preferred source of calories because protein foods are needed for growth and for repair and maintenance of the body, and most protein foods are comparatively expensive. If the diet contains sufficient carbohydrate and fat, the body will not need to rely on protein for calories to produce heat and energy.

It is possible to calculate caloric value of meals if you know the carbohydrate, fat, and protein content of your food. One gram of carbohydrate or protein supplies about four calories; one gram of fat yields nine calories.

If the amount of food you eat contains more calories than you need, the extra calories are stored mainly as fat, and you gain weight. If your caloric intake is insufficient, the body draws from its own reserves to cover the deficit, and you lose weight.

The popular belief that some foods are fattening is not entirely true. Actually any food that adds to your diet more than the required calories is fattening. Highly refined foods add only calories (no minerals or vitamins). Dr. Ruth Leverton calls them "lone-wolf" calories and suggests choosing your calories by the company they keep. Others have referred to them as "empty calories." They could well be omitted from most diets.

Carbohydrates

Carbohydrates, the least expensive sources of calories, supply much of the energy needs. In the form of sugars and starches, they are found in cereals and cereal products, vegetables, legumes, tubers, roots, fruits, honey, sugarcane, sugar beet root, and the sap of maple trees.

Plants use sunlight and chlorophyll to synthesize carbohydrates out of carbon dioxide and water. Humans and animals cannot do this and must eat plants to obtain carbohydrates. The stem, the roots, the leaves, or the seeds of a plant store carbohydrates. When you eat these plant foods, the carbohydrates are changed by digestion into smaller components. Carbohydrates are easily digested and rapidly absorbed into the blood. They are further broken down in the tissues, providing energy for working, eating, sleeping, or just living.

Common carbohydrates in food are sugars, starches, and cellulose. Sugars are composed of one or more simple units called saccharides, while starches and cellulose have hundreds of these saccharide units. Sugars with one unit are called monosaccharides (eg. glucose).

Sucrose (cane, beet, or maple sugar), maltose derived from grains, and lactose in milk have two units and are disaccharides. Starches with their many units are called polysaccharides. When disaccharides and polysaccharides are digested in the body or broken down in the chemistry laboratory, they become monosaccharides or simple sugars.

Carbohydrates are absorbed into the blood from the intestinal tract as monosaccharides and go to the liver to be changed mainly to glucose and glycogen. Glycogen, a polysaccharide, is stored in the body. Glucose is the sugar found in the blood and used by the cells.

You need carbohydrates because they provide the energy for life. In many countries people consider such starchy, high-carbohydrate foods as wheat, rice, corn, oats, or other cereals, and potatoes as the "staff of life." Although the National Research Council does not suggest a definite amount of carbohydrate to be included in the daily diet, forty-five to sixty-five percent of the calories is normal. You can maintain good nutrition on higher or lower amounts if your diet contains fats to provide essential fatty acids, proteins to provide necessary amino acids, and vitamins and minerals.

Because carbohydrates make the diet more palatable, people often feel tempted to eat a large amount of refined carbohydrates, the "empty" calorie foods. These foods, which contribute little or no minerals or vitamins, contain unnecessary calories which may produce unwanted weight gain since the body can convert carbohydrates to fat.

Highly-refined carbohydrate foods such as white sugar, cornstarch, and white flour lost most or all of their vitamin, mineral, and protein content in the milling or refining process. Enrichment, which adds thiamine, riboflavin, niacin, and iron to some cereals, replaces some of the lost vitamins and minerals. Whole grain cereals should be used in preference to "enriched" refined flours, breads, and cereals which do not contain all of the nutrients lost in milling.

Concentrated sweets such as candy, jellies, jams, syrups, and honey may irritate the gastrointestinal tract if eaten in large amounts. They also may impair the appetite for foods high in nutrients. Fresh and dried fruits make better desserts than concentrated sweets, which could well be dispensed with, especially in children's diets.

Cellulose, the chief constituent of the fibrous part of plants, is a carbohydrate not used as fuel by the body because humans lack the enzymes to digest it. But although cellulose provides no calories, it is necessary to the diet because of its regulating function. Cellulose provides bulk or roughage, which stimulates peristaltic movements and prevents constipation. Excess cellulose, however, may lead to other problems, so nutritionists recommend a normal diet which provides a reasonable amount only. The bran fad popular several years ago did considerable damage to some individuals. The best sources of cellulose are raw and cooked vegetables, raw and cooked fruits, legumes, and whole grain cereals.

Fats

Fats are important. They make meals more appetizing and satisfying and, of course, are high in calories. Each gram of fat contains more than twice as many calories as a gram of carbohydrate or protein.

Fat provides insulation and a protective cushion for the organs of your body and a supply of reserve energy. Some oils and fats are carriers of the fat-soluble vitamins and aid in the absorption of these vitamins into the body. A high-fat diet has the connotation of abundance and prosperity. In times of war and famine the conservation of fats is of great concern.

Butter, margarine, shortening, cream, and oil are visible fats. Invisible fats are present in milk, eggs, meats, cheese, nuts, avocados, and olives, and in most other foods in very small amounts.

Today we frequently hear such terms as essential fatty acid, polyunsaturated fat, saturated and unsaturated fat. Fats are composed of glycerol and of units called fatty acids. Certain fatty acids which are needed by the body must be included in the daily diet, since the body cannot manufacture them. These are called essential fatty acids. In experimental work with white rats, lack of essential fatty acids caused poor growth, scaly skin, kidney damage, and inability to reproduce. With the addition of fatty acids to the diet, these symptoms disappeared.

The fatty acid part of the fat is made up of a chain of carbons, like a necklace. Each of the carbons in the chain has two places for hydrogen to be attached. If the carbon chain has all the hydrogen it will hold, the fat is said to be saturated. If some of the carbons do not have hydrogen attached, the fatty acid is unsaturated. A polyunsaturated fatty acid is lacking many hydrogen atoms.

Fats that are liquid at room temperature are known as oils and have a higher proportion of unsaturated fatty acids. Solid fats contain more saturated fatty acids. Animal fats in general and coconut oil have more saturated fatty acids, while vegetable and fish oils contain more of the unsaturated variety.

Nutritionists are giving considerable emphasis to linoleic acid at present. It seems not to be synthesized by the human body and is, therefore, an essential fatty acid. It is also unsaturated. Good sources of linoleic acid are safflower, corn, cottonseed, wheat germ, soybean, and peanut oils. Animal fats contain very little linoleic acid. Ample linoleic acid in the diet is believed to reduce blood cholesterol.

Hydrogenation is widely used in the manufacture of shortenings and margarines to improve the texture, prolong the storage life, and prevent rancidity. This process adds hydrogen to fats. In other words, it changes the unsaturated fatty acids to a saturated form.

On exposure to light and air (oxygen) fats easily become rancid. Moisture and heat hasten this process. Heating fats at high temperatures also leads to undesirable changes. Acrolein, which has a pungent odor, and other irritating substances form when fats are heated to smoking temperatures. Fried foods are undesirable from the standpoint of good nutrition. Particularly harmful is the practice of using fats for frying over and over again.

No optimum allowance has been established for fats in the diet. The recommendations of the Food and Nutrition Board of the National Research Council in 1948 suggested that fat be 20 percent to 25 percent of the total calories of the diet. The average American diet has a much higher percentage of fat than this—40 percent or more of the calories. In this connection, it is noteworthy that Americans have considerably more heart trouble and atherosclerosis than people in countries where the fat consumption is low. In 1963 the Food and Nutrition Board suggested that substituting polyunsaturated for saturated fats is a preventive measure for some individuals. For that reason, there has been much emphasis on polyunsaturated fats.

A relationship seems to exist between the cholesterol levels in the blood with possible atherosclerosis and heart disease, and the quality and quantity of fat as compared with the amount and kind of carbohydrates in the diet. Therefore the following recommendations would be good for most of us: (1) Cut down on the amount of calories from fats and concentrated sweets; (2) Substitute unsaturated fats for at least part of the saturated ones, using more oils to replace some of the solid fats; (3) Reduce the total calories in the diet. In other words, watch the "calorie counters."

Books Which Give Calorie Content and Other Nutritive Values of Foods

Nutritive Value of Foods, Home and Garden Bulletin No. 72, USDA. For sale by the Superintendent of Documents, United States Government Printing Office, Washington, D.C. 20402. Price 25 cents.

Composition of Foods, Agriculture Handbook No. 8, USDA. For sale by the Superintendent of Documents, United States Government Printing Office, Washington, D.C. 20402. Price $1.50.

Food Values of Portions Commonly Used, Bowes and Church; J. B. Lippincott Company, Philadelphia.

The Mine Within You: Minerals

"Eat your spinach, Son. It has minerals in it." Mothers throughout much of the world coax their children to eat with similar statements.

"What's *minerals?*" the child may ask.

"Minerals are . . . well . . . something for your blood. I don't know. Anyway they are good for you." And with that, most mothers feel relieved to let the subject drop.

Of course, the mothers are right. Spinach does contain minerals. And so do bananas, bread, eggs, milk, beans, and most foods. And minerals *are* "good for you." They are essential elements in the blood—and in the nerves, muscles, and other tissues. They build bones and teeth. Other functions are coming to be understood, but much still remains to be learned about minerals. One thing is certain: they are essential.

If you could extract all of the minerals from your body, you would have a heap weighing about six and a half pounds. It would consist mostly of calcium and phosphorus, with some magnesium, sodium, potassium, iron, iodine, and about twenty other minerals, some in such minute amounts that they are called "trace elements."

The minerals found in the body are sometimes grouped as macrominerals (calcium, phosphorus, magnesium, potassium, sodium, chlorine, sulfur) and microminerals (iron, manganese, copper, and iodine). In addition some of the trace elements are known to be essential for body functions (cobalt, fluorine, zinc, selenium, molybdenum), some appear to be essential (chromium), but the functions of some are not known (aluminum, arsenic, boron, bromine, cadmium, lead, nickel, silicon, strontium, vanadium).

Calcium makes up about half of the body's six and one half pounds of minerals, and phosphorus about one-fourth. The remaining macrominerals together account for another pound and a half. The microminerals, mostly iron, weigh little more than one-tenth of an ounce.

The bones and teeth contain the bulk of the body's minerals, but minerals are essential in other parts of the body too. Thyroxin contains iodine, vitamin B_{12} contains cobalt, hemoglobin has iron, and so on.

Calcium and Phosphorus. The skeleton, the framework to which muscles are attached making movement possible, is composed principally of three minerals: calcium, phosphorus, and magnesium. Teeth are built of the same materials.

The teeth and bones contain 99 percent of the calcium and 70 to 80 percent of the phosphorus in the body, so these minerals are sometimes classed together. The National Research Council recommends the same allowances for both except during the first year of life.

Calcium and phosphorus are not the only nutrients essential to bones and teeth, however. Magnesium, fluorine, manganese, vitamins A, C, and D, and even protein are all in some way involved.

Calcium is also needed for muscles, nerves, blood clotting, and some enzyme activity. Yet calcium is a most frequently lacking nutrient in United States diets. No wonder adults, as well as children, are encouraged to drink milk, since it has a high content of calcium easily utilized by the body. One cup of milk furnishes about 280 milligrams of calcium. Two cups a day with an otherwise adequate diet, should provide for adult needs.

Other foods which are good to fair sources of calcium are milk products, greens (including collards, dandelion, kale, mustard, and turnips), other vegetables, some fruits and nuts, and most of the legumes.

You may have heard that some foods are "calcium robbers." It is true that chard, beet greens, spinach, and rhubarb contain oxalic acid which forms an insoluble salt with calcium, but these foods are not usually eaten in great quantities. And they are believed not to affect the calcium utilization of other foods eaten at the same meal;

therefore they are really not important in connection with calcium. Something important to note, however, is that rhubarb leaves contain high concentrations of oxalic acid and some other deleterious substances. They should never be eaten, since they are not safe, even in small amounts.

Whole wheat and other whole grain cereals contain phytic acid which binds calcium so that it apparently is not absorbed. However, Drs. Wohl and Goodhart* point out that the body must be able under some circumstances to adapt to high intakes of phytic acid since whole tribes have lived in apparent health using enough whole wheat theorically to cause a loss of more calcium than consumed.

Phosphorus might be described as one of the busiest minerals. It is an essential factor in the metabolism of carbohydrates, fats, and proteins, is part of the buffer system that maintains the body's acid-base balance, is in the cytoplasm of all cells, and is a part of the genes that transmit hereditary characteristics. All this and more is in addition to its functions in the bones and teeth.

The diet will probably have sufficient phosphorus if calcium and protein needs are met. The recommended allowance for phosphorus is the same as for calcium, 800 milligrams a day for adults with additional amounts during pregnancy and lactation, and with varying allowances for children depending upon age.

Among the good food sources of phosphorus are milk and milk products; dried beans, peas, and other legumes; nuts, especially peanuts and brazil nuts; oatmeal and other whole grain cereals; eggs; meats; fish; and fowl.

Vitamin D, formed in the skin by the action of sunshine, is essential for the absorption of calcium and phosphorus. Normally the calcium in the body is maintained in balance between the bony tissues and fluids by two hormones, parathormone and calcitonin, aided by vitamin D.

Without sufficient vitamin D, calcium, and phosphorus, a child may develop the soft, bowed bones of rickets, a condition frequently observed in places with little sunshine. In these areas children may be given vitamin D preparations, cod or other fish liver oils. An adult form of rickets, osteomalacia, was common in purdah women in India

*Michael G. Wohl and Robert S. Goodhart, *Modern Nutrition in Health and Disease,* fourth edition, Lea and Febiger, 1968.

and Mohammedan lands who were confined indoors without benefit of sunlight.

Magnesium. Your body normally contains about an ounce of magnesium, which cooperates with calcium and phosphorus to form bones and teeth. Magnesium is also important to the heart, nerves, and muscles.

Alcoholics may have low levels of magnesium, but normal people seldom suffer from magnesium deficiency since it is widely available in foods. The National Research Council recommends a magnesium allowance of 300-400 milligrams daily for adults, increased to 450 milligrams during pregnancy and lactation, and amounts varying with age in infancy and childhood.

Magnesium is found in largest quantity in nuts, whole grains, beans, peas, soybeans, and in green leafy vegetables since it is part of the structure of chlorophyll.

Iron. The three grams of iron in your body would be enough to make only a small nail, but this mininutrient does maximum work.

The liver and spleen store approximately one gram of iron. The rest is in the hemoglobin, in the myoglobin of muscles, and in various enzymes.

Throughout life the body continually needs iron, although it uses and reuses every bit it gets. Children and teen-agers need comparatively more iron than adults. Women during pregnancy and lactation, in fact through the child-bearing years, have a high requirement. Their recommended allowance (18 milligrams a day) is nearly twice the 10 milligrams recommended for men.

Sufficient iron to meet the recommended allowances for women is frequently not included in the average diet. However, by taking care to choose foods rich in iron daily, a woman can avoid anemia due to iron deficiency.

Among the good iron sources are egg yolk, whole wheat, nuts, dates, dried fruits, beans, lentils, green leafy vegetables, oatmeal, liver, molasses, and meats.

Iodine. Not many years ago iodine deficiency became recognized as a public health problem. Simple goiter, which is an enlargement of the thyroid gland in the neck, was common; and it was found to be caused by lack of sufficient iodine in the food. Goiter was observed especially among people who lived far from the sea, as in the Great

Lakes region in the United States, the Alpine mountains in Europe, or the Andean plateaus of South America.

With the addition of a small amount of iodine to table salt, simple goiter can be largely eradicated. Those living near the sea, eating sea foods, or those using iodized salt get enough iodine to meet the recommended daily allowances of 80 to 140 micrograms for adults. The allowances for children vary with age and sex.

Fluorine. Recently it has been discovered that adequate fluorine helps to maintain strong bones and to prevent dental caries (cavities). It appears that it may be beneficial in osteoporosis, a demineralization of the bones, usually observed in older persons.

Since dental caries are rampant in the United States, fluoridation of water has been suggested and is a subject of considerable controversy.

The addition of fluorine to water of low fluorine content has appeared to result in fewer dental caries. The amount that will protect teeth from caries is one to one and a half parts of fluorine per million parts of water. In concentrations higher than 1.5 parts per million, mottling of the teeth may result. Where water has excessive fluorine as in the Texas Panhandle and in certain regions of Colorado, mottling of the teeth is quite common among residents.

Copper. Copper helps to form hemoglobin although it is not a part of it. Copper is found in certain enzymes and ceruloplasmin, a protein in the blood.

If the diet is adequate in other respects, it should provide sufficient copper.

Cobalt. Cobalt is a part of vitamin B_{12}, and its function is linked to that of the vitamin.

Cattle and other ruminants can form their own vitamin B_{12} if their feed contains sufficient cobalt. If pastures lack cobalt, these animals become anemic and have other symptoms that can be cured by adding either vitamin B_{12} or cobalt to the feed.

Humans cannot synthesize vitamin B_{12} in their tissues, so they must take it in their food. Since cobalt is at the core of vitamin B_{12}, sufficient vitamin B_{12} in the diet assures sufficient cobalt. Vitamin B_{12} has been called the "animal protein factor" because it is found almost exclusively in animal foods. Vegetable foods either do not have any or have very negligible amounts.

Zinc. Only minute quantities of zinc are found in the body, but it has important functions. Its highest concentrations are in the bones, skin, liver, and blood. It is involved in a number of enzyme systems and has been found to promote wound healing. Authorities in Iran and Egypt have reported an anemia accompanied by dwarfism and attributed to zinc deficiency.

The usual dietary includes ten to fifteen milligrams of zinc. Zinc can be toxic and cause poisoning if taken in too large amounts. It is widely distributed in foods, so there is ordinarily little chance of lack in the diet. Best sources are wheat germ, yeast, liver, and sea foods.

Sodium, Potasium, and Chlorine. These minerals help to maintain the acid-base balance and have other essential functions. They are in adequate supply in the average diet.

Selenium, Manganese, Molybdenum. Selenium, known as "factor 3," is associated with vitamin E functions. Animals of some species have been found to require selenium, but too much can be toxic. "Blind staggers" is due to selenium poisoning and may occur when animals graze on alkali pastures.

Manganese and molybdenum assist certain enzymes at their work.

Acid-base Balance. If a person comes to your door selling "alkalizing" concoctions, watch out. What you buy may be more harmful than helpful. You may have heard that there are acid-forming foods and alkaline-forming foods. You may have been told that you must beware of acid-forming foods, and so perhaps you feel somewhat apprehensive.

Actually the body has ways in which to maintain the delicate balance between the acids and bases formed in the utilization of foods. When you burn wood in your fireplace, ashes are left. When food is eaten, we speak of its being burned in the body and forming an ash or residue.

For instance if you were to burn cereals, cheese, eggs, meats, fish, poultry, walnuts, peanuts, filberts, Brazil nuts, lentils, macaroni, and noodles in the laboratory, they would leave an ash residue. On analysis the ash would be found to have an excess of phosphorus, sulfur, and chlorine. They are components of an acid ash, therefore these foods are said to leave acid residues.

On the other hand if vegetables, potatoes, fruits, milk, molasses, legumes, and some nuts were burned, these ashes would contain an excess of calcium, potassium, sodium, and magnesium. These foods, and others that may have an acid taste, leave an alkaline or base ash.

Here is the way in which the body acts when confronted with an excess of either acid or alkaline residue. The body contains substances called buffers which can combine with either acids or bases. If excess acid is formed, buffers neutralize it. If the excess is base, buffers neutralize it also.

If the body has too much acid, the kidneys will normally make the urine more acid and thus eliminate the excess. The same is true with an excess base. The buffers, the kidneys, and the lungs will, under normal conditions, neutralize the acids and bases. In this way the blood and other fluids are maintained in a slightly alkaline state.

A food's being an acid- or alkaline-ash yielder has nothing to do with its taste. For instance, orange juice tastes acid because of the organic acids in it. But these acids usually combine with basic substances leaving an alkaline ash in the body. Cereals and meat, which do not taste acid, render acid ash.

A normally healthy person who eats an adequate diet with a variety of fruits and vegetables, milk products, cereals, and protein foods, does not need to concern himself about the body's acid-base balance. It works automatically.

Water

When Sir Edmund Hillary and his expedition first reached the summit of Mount Everest in 1953, it was said that an adequate water supply was the greatest factor in their success. Other expeditions before theirs had not made proper provision for water to balance the losses, and the climbers had to return, their goal not reached.

"The sea within us," as one author puts it, accounts for more than half the body weight of an adult person. We may go without food for weeks, but we can go only a few days without water. It has been suggested by nutrition scientists that a person may lose all his glycogen, all his fat, and half his protein without real danger, but losing just 10 percent of his body water is serious, and 20 to 22 percent is fatal.

Water may escape from the body through the lungs, the kidneys, the skin, and the gastrointestinal tract. These losses must be constantly replenished.

Why is water so important? Simply because it has so many jobs to do. Water is part of every cell. It transports all the foodstuffs to the cells, and the operations within the cells occur in a watery medium. Substances in the body have to be maintained in solution, and secretions and wastes must be carried out of the cells by water. Water regulates the body temperature, adjusting to the water losses and the changes in the surroundings. Four quarts of water are constantly circulating in the body as part of the blood.

Children lose water easily since their bodies contain proportionately more water than adults, and they have comparatively larger surface areas and higher metabolic rates. Thus an infant or a child has to drink water more often. Dehydration may occur very quickly if a child vomits or has diarrhea or is exposed to too much heat.

In hot weather or while driving through the desert be sure to have plenty of water to drink. If you do hard work in hot surroundings, not only water but also salt should be replenished if the loss is persistent.

Six to eight glasses of fluid a day is recommended. When you get up in the morning try drinking a glass or more of fresh water. It will perk you up and start your day well.

The Vital Sparks: Vitamins

Although less than a hundred years ago nobody had ever heard of a "vitamin," the word today is a common household term, and mothers worry frequently that their children are not consuming enough of them. Americans spend millions of dollars annually for vitamin concentrates. Many, concerned that their food pattern or that of their family lacks certain vitamins, cling to these vitamin or vitamin-mineral concentrates as a vital part of their diet. Yet despite all the concern and money spent on vitamins today, it was not until 1911 that anybody isolated vitamins and recognized the vital functions they perform in the body.

The story of the discovery of vitamins is as fascinating as detective fiction. The results of their deficiency in the diet have been observed for thousands of years. Yet through the centuries no one conceived the idea that lack of various substances in food could actually cause disease or, when present, prevent it. So vitamins, though as old as life, are yet as modern as the twentieth century.

For hundreds of years explorers and ship's crews on long voyages developed scurvy, a disease known as the "scourge of the sea." More sailors succumbed to it than to sea warfare and accidents combined. Scurvy also followed wars and famines on land. But only two hundred years ago did a doctor in the British navy discover that limes and lemons cured the disease. Limes and other citrus fruits were added to the navy rations, and British sailors came to be called "Limeys," a name which still sticks.

Here and there around the world other pieces of evidence contributed to the vitamin story. A Dutch physician in Java, an exiled Polish doctor, a Cambridge professor, a Japanese navy doctor—all added their bit to the detection of the cause of beriberi, another disease caused by lack of a vitamin. Beriberi mostly afflicted people in rice-eating countries.

Still another vitamin deficiency disease, pellagra, was observed largely in corn-eating communities.

Children who had little access to sunshine or fish liver oils developed rickets, because they lacked yet another vitamin.

Jean Dumas, a Frenchman, is credited with being the first scientist to suggest that the diet required something other than protein, fat, and carbohydrate. His observation came in 1870, when food was scarce during the Franco-Prussian War. Artificial milk prepared of purified protein, fat, carbohydrate, and salts was fed to infants and children with tragic results. Scientist Dumas pointed out that there must be some still unknown essential factor.

Although these and other scattered bits of evidence accumulated in the eighteenth and nineteenth centuries, the most significant discoveries about vitamins were left for the twentieth century. Still to be accomplished was the recognition, isolation, and synthesis of the amazing and indispensable substances that can make the difference between life and death.

In 1911 Casimir Funk, a Polish chemist, introduced the word "vitamine." He believed that vitamins were vital to life and that they were amines. Other scientists had referred to them as "accessory food factors," but Dr. Funk related them to scurvy, pellagra, rickets, and beriberi, which he properly labeled deficiency diseases. Later when the chemical nature of the various vitamins became known, the "e" was dropped, and the name became "vitamin."

Vitamins are defined as "organic substances occurring in natural foods, required in minute amounts by the body for normal nutrition and health." They neither furnish energy nor are they a part of the body tissues, but life depends on them. They are involved in the action of enzymes and in many other body processes. They are the vital sparks.

In addition to the vitamins supplied in our food, at least one, niacin, is formed in the body from an amino acid, tryptophan. Some vitamins may be manufactured by action of certain bacteria in the intestines.

In the order of their discovery, vitamins were assigned letter names. Vitamin A was the first one recognized, followed by vitamin B, vitamin C, and so on. Today names related to the chemical nature of the vitamins are preferred, such as thiamin for vitamin B_1, riboflavin for vitamin B_2, and ascorbic acid for vitamin C.

Vitamins are divided into two groups: those soluble in fats and fat solvents, and those soluble in water. The fat-soluble vitamins A, D, E, and K are absorbed in the body with the fats. When something hinders fat absorption, the utilization of the fat-soluble vitamins is affected.

The water-soluble vitamins include vitamin C and the vitamin B complex. The water-soluble group is easily lost during cooking, especially if considerable water is used and discarded. Some vitamins are destroyed by heat, others by light and air, and some by alkalies, such as baking soda. Some are affected by all these factors. To avoid heavy vitamin losses follow good cooking practices.

Scurvy, beriberi, pellagra, and rickets have been largely eradicated in the United States and other developed countries, but vitamin deficiency diseases are still a possibility even in these countries. Special care needs to be employed to provide everyone, particularly infants, growing children, adolescents, pregnant and nursing women, and elderly people, with a nourishing diet. An adequate diet with ample minerals and vitamins includes such basic foods as milk and milk products, protein-rich foods, fresh fruits and vegetables, and various kinds of whole grain or enriched breads and cereals.

The question sometimes is asked, and it is a pertinent one, "Can you take too many vitamins?" This is very unlikely if you get them as they come naturally in food. However, large dosages of the fat-soluble vitamins A and D may produce toxic effects. Concentrates of water-soluble vitamins are not usually toxic because the body excretes the excess.

It is wise to consult a physician before using supplementary vitamins, especially before dosing small children with them. A good varied diet remains the best source of vitamins, in which case danger of either overconsumption or lack of vitamins rarely occurs. Unfortunately, even in the United States with its abundance of food, many people are not eating an adequate diet.

The Fat-soluble Vitamins

Vitamin A. Vitamin A, whose chemical name is retinol, was the first vitamin to be labeled. It is essential for growth and reproduction, which can be said of many vitamins. It helps to maintain healthy skin and mucous membranes, safeguarding the body against bacteria and infection.

Vitamin A is needed for healthy eyes. It has on occasion been referred to as the "antixerophthalmic factor" because xerophthalmia or "dry eye" was the first disease associated with a vitamin A deficiency. If not treated, xerophthalmia, still prevalent in many parts of the world, causes blindness. An estimated 80,000 children under four become blind annually because of lack of vitamin A.

The retina of the eye contains a pigment, rhodopsin or visual purple, formed from protein and vitamin A. Visual purple builds up in dim light and breaks down in bright light. If sufficient vitamin A is not supplied, regeneration does not take place normally. The result is poor adaptation to the dark, and impaired night vision, called night blindness.

While vitamin A as such is found only in animal foods, it can also be obtained by choosing vegetable foods containing carotene, a substance which the body converts to vitamin A. Utilization of vitamin A in the body is influenced by a number of factors: (1) Conversion of carotene to vitamin A is affected by thyroxin and the amount and kind of protein. (2) Absorption of vitamin A requires bile salts and normal structure and function of the small intestines. In ulcerative colitis, diarrhea, and some other conditions, absorption is hindered. Cooking vegetables improves the body's utilization of the carotene in them. (3) Destruction of vitamin A by oxygen may be counteracted by natural antioxidants, such as vitamin E. Ninety percent of the vitamin A in the body is stored in the liver.

The World Health Organization has adopted international units (I.U.) of measurement for vitamin A and carotene and other vitamins. If one relies on carotene as the principal source of the vitamin, he must provide large amounts, since two I.U. of carotene are equal to one I.U. of vitamin A. Dr. LeRoy Voris, executive secretary of the Food and Nutrition Board, National Research Council of the National Academy of Sciences, states that the average household diet in the United States provides about 7500 I.U., about one half of it derived from carotene.

The daily amount recommended by the Food and Nutrition Board (referred to as the Recommended Dietary Allowances, or RDA) is 5000 I.U. for adults, 6000 I.U. during pregnancy, and 8000 I.U. during lactation. Children's allowances vary with age. Note page 149. This allowance assumes that part of the vitamin is in the form of carotene. It is not based on minimum need but is "adequate to meet the needs of health." Excessive amounts of vitamin A have caused toxic symptoms in both adults and children.

The amount of both vitamin A and carotene in the same type food varies. For example, summer milk may contain twice as much vitamin A as winter milk. Carotene in vegetables such as carrots may vary from 2200 to 47,000 I.U. per scant half cup, and dark green leafy vegetables from 6000 to 12,000 I.U., according to some chemical determinations.

The best sources of vitamin A and carotene are fish liver oils, liver, butter, margarine, cream, egg yolk, most green leafy and yellow vegetables, fresh and dried apricots, cantaloupes, and persimmons. Good sources are whole milk, cheese, peaches, prunes, papayas, tomatoes.

Vitamin D. Vitamin D, termed the antirachitic factor, is essential for prevention of rickets, for normal growth, and for proper formation of bones and teeth. It aids in the absorption of calcium and phosphorus.

Rickets, caused largely by lack of vitamin D, is characterized by poorly calcified bones. Rickets is seldom seen in the tropics and subtropics where sunshine is plentiful the year around. But the condition can still be found in rainy and cloudy parts of the world. It was widespread in parts of the United States before the discovery of vitamin D. But now the common practices of irradiating milk and adding vitamin D to other foods make it very unlikely for vitamin D deficiency to occur in the United States, except in extremely deprived areas.

Children are most affected by lack of vitamin D, but a form of adult rickets, called osteomalacia, afflicts confined individuals and some Oriental women who, according to custom, remain indoors or go outdoors only with veiled faces and almost totally covered bodies.

Most food does not contain significant amounts of vitamin D. Notable exceptions are cod liver oil and some other fish liver oils. Milk, liver, and egg yolk are fair sources.

But the body possesses a marvelous compensatory mechanism. Beneath the skin is a form of cholesterol. When irradiated with ultraviolet light from sunshine, the cholesterol changes into vitamin D and thus acquires antirachitic properties. Unfortunately, glass, fog, smog, clouds, and dust may filter out these rays and hinder the formation of vitamin D. Another source of vitamin D is a compound found in plants and yeast. When irradiated, it may be transformed into vitamin D.

The RDA for vitamin D is 400 I.U. daily for infants, children, adolescents, and pregnant and nursing mothers. No recommended allowances are made for other adults after the age of twenty-two years.

It is wise not to overdo vitamin consumption. Excessive intake of vitamin D retards growth and may cause anemia and produce toxic effects. Common symptoms are anorexia (loss of appetite), vomiting, headache, drowsiness, and diarrhea.

Vitamin E. It has been said that vitamin E is a vitamin looking for a disease. The book *Human Nutrition and Dietetics** speaks of it as "one of those embarrassing vitamins." Vitamin E was discovered, identified, named tocopherol, and synthesized years ago, but many questions remain unanswered regarding its functions in the human body. However, it is known to be an essential dietary factor, and its need by animals has long been recognized.

Vitamin E was first called the reproductive vitamin because it was found to affect reproduction in some animals. This was not a good designation, however, because other vitamins are also essential for reproduction, and vitamin E does not appear to influence human reproduction in any striking way.

It is an important antioxidant in the body. As such it protects vitamin A and polyunsaturated fatty acids from oxidation. In recent years many people have substituted polyunsaturated fatty acids for other fats in an effort to lower their cholesterol level. This increased use of polyunsaturated fats increases the need for vitamin E in the diet.

Vitamin E is essential for the structure and function of living cells and appears to play some role in enzyme systems and in the

---

*Stanley Davidson and R. Passmore, *Human Nutrition and Dietetics,* Williams and Wilkins, Baltimore, 1963.

formation of red blood cells. Research designed to learn more about the function of this interesting vitamin is currently in process.

Although the function of vitamin E in the human body is not yet fully established, the 1968 National Research Council revision, page 16, includes RDA for vitamin E from infancy through old age. The adult RDA is 30 I.U. for men and pregnant and lactating women and 25 I.U. for other women.

Vitamin E is stable to heat but readily destroyed by oxidation, ultraviolet light, some iron salts, and rancid fats. It is widely distributed in foods, so under normal conditions there is little possibility of a lack. The richest dietary sources are oils of cotton seed, other seeds, wheat germ, rice germ, peanuts, corn, and soybeans. Fair sources are dark green leafy vegetables, eggs, nuts, legumes, and whole grain cereals.

Vitamin K. Vitamin K is essential for normal blood clotting and recent research suggests other functions. A deficiency of this vitamin results in man from either faulty absorption or liver disorders.

Consuming large amounts of sulfa drugs or antibiotics may interfere with the normal production of vitamin K by destroying the bacteria in the intestines which produce the vitamin.

Normally, little likelihood exists of a lack of vitamin K caused by faulty nutrition since it is produced in the intestines and widely distributed in foods. The best food sources are green leafy vegetables, alfalfa, cauliflower, cabbage, and soybean oil.

Water-soluble Vitamins

Vitamin C (Ascorbic Acid). Vitamin C, now generally known by its chemical name, ascorbic acid, has been called the vitamin of fresh fruits and vegetables. The effects of its lack have been known since ancient times. The disease described in a papyrus, believed to have been written about 1,500 years before Christ, might have been scurvy. This vitamin C deficiency disease, feared for centuries by sailors, causes spongy and bleeding gums, hemorrhages under the skin, and great weakness. Death follows if vitamin C is not given. While scurvy today is rare, there still exists what are termed "subclinical symptoms" of vitamin C deficiency.

Ascorbic acid may be a factor in the body's reaction to stress. It appears to play a vital role in certain body enzyme systems, activity of the vitamin folic acid, and the metabolism of some amino acids, and aids in the absorption of iron from the intestines. It is essential for healthy bones and teeth and strong capillary walls and appears to be involved in some way in resisting infection.

Man, monkeys, guinea pigs, the Indian fruit bat, and the red-vented bulbul are the only creatures known that must rely on food as the source of ascorbic acid. Most animals manufacture their own.

Ascorbic acid requirements are on a daily basis, since this vitamin is not stored in the body to any great extent and what is not used is largely excreted. The recommended daily dietary allowances for adults are 55 milligrams for women, and 60 milligrams for men and for pregnant and nursing women. The allowances for children are somewhat less, depending on age. One half glass of orange juice, two thirds glass of grapefruit juice, or one and a half glasses of tomato juice will provide the day's requirement.

Among the best sources of ascorbic acid are citrus fruits (lemons, limes, oranges, grapefruit, tangerines), berries, cantaloupes and other melons, greens, green peppers, cabbage, Brussels sprouts, broccoli, tomatoes, rose hips. Some tropical fruits are excellent sources, especially the acerola or West Indies cherry, the richest known source.

Ascorbic acid is very unstable and easily lost during storage, processing, or cooking. Light hastens its inactivation, and so does air. Enzymes in harvested foods may destroy the vitamin. To avoid this, vegetables which are to be frozen should be first blanched. Soaking or cooking water can dissolve ascorbic acid, and frequently does.

Commercial food processors take precautions in canning, drying, and freezing of foods to avoid, as much as possible, the losses of ascorbic acid during storage, processing, or cooking. Frozen and commercially canned and freeze-dried fruits and vegetables usually retain a high percentage of the vitamin. Similar care may be taken at home to preserve ascorbic acid. Fresh foods should be stored at low temperatures, away from contact with light and air.

Fruits with strong skins, root vegetables, or those with tight leaves such as cabbage, lose ascorbic acid more slowly. Cooking vegetables in small amounts of water and avoiding overcooking and reheating, when possible, help to retain vitamin C. Copper tends to destroy ascorbic acid; therefore exposed copper kettles are not recommended. While soda maintains the green color of vegetables, it destroys ascorbic acid and other vitamins; so its use should be avoided.

The B Vitamins.

Thiamin (Vitamin B_1). Thiamin was originally called the antineuritic factor or antiberiberi vitamin. It is necessary for normal growth and for the metabolism of carbohydrates. While today pronounced deficiency states are not often observed, mild deficiencies due to low thiamin intake are fairly common. Some of the symptoms are loss of appetite, constipation, fatigue, and nervousness.

The RDA for thiamin is based on the calories in the diet and assumes moderate activity. For each 1,000 calories, a minimum of 0.5 milligram is recommended. If a person is on a reducing diet or for any reason consumes less than 2,000 calories, however, the amount of thiamin should be no less than 1.0 milligram daily. The 1968 NRC Revision increased somewhat the RDA for thiamin. The requirements for children vary with age. The adult allowances range from 1.0 for women over eighteen years of age to 1.5 milligrams for boys fourteen to eighteen years. During pregnancy 0.1 milligram is added to the basic requirements, and 0.5 milligram during lactation.

Thiamin is widely distributed in foods. Richest sources are germ of cereals, brewers' yeast, whole grain cereals, fresh green vegetables, nuts, and legumes. Such food items as fats, oils, sugar, and sulfured dried fruits are nearly, if not entirely, devoid of thiamin. Milling of grains removes thiamin, which is concentrated in the bran and the germ. Enrichment programs, which restore some of the nutrients removed by milling, have improved the nutrition of many individuals. Such programs enrich hulled rice in Oriental countries and milled corn and wheat in the United States.

Thiamin is easily destroyed by heat, especially in alkaline solutions such as with soda. Some of the vitamin is lost in roasting and baking and the overcooking of foods. When you discard the cooking water of vegetables, you are throwing away the thiamin and other vitamins which the vegetables contained.

Riboflavin (Vitamin B_2). Riboflavin, like most of the vitamins, is necessary for normal growth and development. It combines with other nutrients to form enzymes involved in the processes of living cells.

Riboflavin helps to maintain the eyes in a healthy state. Itching, burning eyes, a sandy feeling, eyestrain, and sensitivity to light are some of the symptoms of deficiency. Cheilosis is another symptom. In this condition the lips split at the angles of the mouth, and the tongue becomes sore and red. Dermatitis of a fatty kind is seen sometimes on the face, especially around the nose and ears.

Riboflavin requirements are related to caloric intake and protein needs. Adult men need an average daily amount of 1.7 milligrams and women of 1.5 milligrams. This increases during pregnancy to 1.8 milligrams and during lactation to 2.0 milligrams.

Riboflavin is stable to heat but is destroyed by exposure to sunlight. It is widely distributed, though frequently in small amounts, in animal and vegetable foods. Best sources are milk, liver, brewers' yeast, cheese, eggs, green leafy vegetables, whole grain or enriched cereals and flour, lean meat, legumes, and nuts.

Niacin. Although niacin was prepared in the chemical laboratory a hundred years ago, it was many years before it was recognized as a vitamin and a pellagra preventive factor. Pellagra was a dreaded disease in the southern part of the United States. It was termed the disease of the "3 D's"—diarrhea, dermatitis, and dementia. A fourth D—death—often followed before niacin was discovered to prevent and cure pellagra.

Dr. Joseph Goldberger, studying the problem of pellagra in the South from 1912 to 1928, noticed a relationship between diet and pellagra. He recommended changes in the diet of asylums, orphanages, and state prisons where pellagra was rampant. At one time as many as 200,000 people were suffering with pellagra in the United States, and many of them died. Dr. Goldberger also conducted experiments on dogs. He produced blacktongue in them by feeding them diets similar to that of pellagra patients. He even discovered that a substance in yeast would prevent the condition, but he did not live to see the unraveling of the cause of the disease and its cure with niacin.

In 1937 Conrad Elvehjem and his associates cured blacktongue in dogs with nicotinic acid or nicotinamide. When niacin, the name preferred in the United States for this substance, was prescribed for pellagra patients, dramatic cures resulted. During World War II a good diet was emphasized and the enrichment program was begun. Enrichment of cereal and flour added niacin along with thiamin, riboflavin, and iron. After the war pellagra almost ceased to exist, and today is said to be a clinical curiosity in the United States.

Pellagra has been considered a disease of the corn-eating areas of the world, but recent reports indicate that pellagra also commonly afflicts the poor in Hyderabad, India. There the main staple in the diet is not corn but a millet called jowar.

Willard Krehl and his associates discovered in 1945 that niacin could be formed from tryptophan, an essential amino acid. This process is accelerated by vitamin B_6. Sixty milligrams of tryptophan furnish one milligram of niacin. Thus niacin equivalents include, in addition to dietary niacin, 1 milligram equivalent for each sixty milligrams of dietary tryptophan.

Recommended daily allowances of niacin vary with age and sex. For men the RDA is 18 milligram equivalents, for women 13 milligram equivalents, during pregnancy 15 milligram equivalents, and during lactation 20 milligram equivalents.

Best food sources of niacin are peanuts, yeast, liver, meats, fish, legumes, whole grains, most dried fruits, and some nuts.

Vitamin B_6. The need for vitamin B_6 by humans was discovered by chance comparatively recently when babies fed a commercial liquid formula developed severe symptoms, which were cured with vitamin B_6.

Vitamin B_6 is not a single unit but three closely related compounds: pyridoxine from vegetable sources and pyridoxal and pyridoxamine from animal sources. They all have similar effects in the body.

Vitamin B_6 appears to be essential to good health. It is involved in the production of niacin from tryptophan and in the metabolism of carbohydrates, polyunsaturated fatty acids, and proteins.

Following exposure to radiation, in tuberculosis after dosage with some drugs, in old age, and during pregnancy, especially with severe nausea and vomiting, extra amounts of vitamin B_6 seem to be beneficial.

Because vitamin B_6 is found in a wide variety of foods, deficiency of the vitamin is not common under ordinary circumstances. Weakness, loss of appetite, soreness of lips and tongue, oily dermatitis, insomnia, nervousness, irritability, kidney stones, and anemia which does not respond to iron therapy are some of the reported deficiency symptoms.

Vitamin B_6 appears for the first time in the NRC 1968 revision of the Recommended Daily Dietary Allowances. The adult RDA is 2.0 milligrams with 2.5 milligrams during pregnancy and lactation. Ordinary diets are said to provide between 1 and 3 milligrams.

Best dietary sources are wheat germ, bran, whole grain cereals, liver, soybeans, split peas, bananas, avocados, peanuts, some dried fruits, and meat. Vitamin B_6 is destroyed by light and to some extent by cooking. Considerable food value is lost in milling and is not replaced by enrichment.

Vitamin B_{12} (Cobalamin). Vitamin B_{12} is one of the most recently recognized vitamins, having been discovered in 1948. It contains cobalt and was therefore given the chemical name cobalamin. It seems to be associated with folacin. It is chiefly known in its relation to pernicious anemia and the formation of red blood cells, but it appears to be essential for the function of all the body cells.

Since vitamin B_{12} is very potent, the body seems to require only minute amounts. The RDA is 5 micrograms per day for adults to age fifty-five. After that age the amount is increased to 6 micrograms. In pregnancy it is 8 micrograms and during lactation, 6 micrograms. It is estimated that only about 30 percent of vitamin B_{12} in food is absorbed by normal individuals.

Vitamin B_{12} is produced by microorganisms such as bacteria and fungi. It seems to be found almost exclusively in animal foods. The moderate use of milk and eggs in the diet insures an adequate amount.

It should be noted that evaporated milk and yogurt have been found to be very poor sources. A considerable amount of vitamin B_{12} is destroyed by heat.

Folacin (Folic Acid). Folacin (from the Latin word for leaf) is a vitamin of many names. Besides folacin, folic acid, folate, and its chemical name pteroylglutamic acid (PGA), it has been called vitamin B_c, vitamin M, vitamin U, lacto-bacillus casei factor, and citrovorum factor. Folacin is the name favored by the National Research Council.

It is essential for growth and reproduction and is involved in various metabolic processes, especially with amino acids. It is associated with hemoglobin formation and prevention of certain types of anemia. It appears to have some connection with the functions of vitamin B_{12}, ascorbic acid, iron, and some hormones.

Folacin is synthesized in the intestines of some animals but apparently man has to depend upon food as a source. A deficiency is not likely, though, except during pregnancy and infancy, and in certain disease conditions.

The NRC 1968 revision has included allowances for folacin. They are 0.4 milligrams a day for adults, increased to 0.8 milligrams in pregnancy and 0.5 milligrams during lactation.

Folacin is quite widely distributed in foods. Deep green leafy vegetables, yeast, and liver are the best sources and whole wheat cereals, dried legumes, and nuts are good sources. Storage at room temperature and cooking at high temperatures cause loss of folacin.

Other Vitamins

There are other vitamins which are known to be essential for health for which no recommended daily dietary allowances are suggested. This does not mean that they are unimportant. It may be because no clear-cut dietary deficiencies have been established, there are liberal amounts in common foods, or not sufficient is known to determine a requirement for humans.

Pantothenic acid is an important part of coenzyme A and is involved in the metabolism of the major nutrients. Biotin is essential for the transfer of a one-carbon group to form malonyl coenzyme A, a substance very much needed for the formation of fatty acids. There are other vitamins and vitamin-like substances such as choline, inositol, and para-amino benzoic acid.

In Summary

Vitamins—the vital sparks—are essential substances for life and health along with proteins, carbohydrates, fats, and minerals. The nutrients interact, and the lack of one may affect the requirements or the functions of others. An adequate intake of all of them in everyday foods is essential for buoyant health. Unrefined foods probably contain as yet undiscovered vitamins which we will hear about in years to come.

FAT-SOLUBLE VITAMINS

Names	Functions in the Body	Some Symptoms of Deficiency
Vitamin A Retinol Provitamin: Carotene	Promotes normal growth and tissue repair. Maintains healthy eyes and normal vision. Protects against infection by promoting health of skin and mucous membrane. Aids normal bone development and tooth formation.	Retarded growth. Faulty bone and teeth development. Dry, rough, scaly skin. Night blindness. Glare blindness. Xerophthalmia. Large amts. are toxic.
Vitamin D Vitamin D_2 Calciferol Viosterol Ergosterol Vitamin D_3	Essential for normal growth and development and formation of bones and teeth. Aids in absorption of calcium and phosphorus. Prevents and cures rickets and osteomalacia. Stored largely in liver.	Rickets. Osteomalacia. Poor teeth. Large amts. are toxic.
Vitamin E Tocopherols	Essential for structure and function of living cells and formation of blood cells. Is antioxidant and assists in preventing oxidation of polyunsaturated fatty acids and vitamin A. Interrelated with selenium. Not stored in body to any extent.	In humans, not as yet determined. Mild anemia.
Vitamin K Menadione	Involved in formation of prothrombin and normal blood clotting.	Slow blood clotting time. Hemorrhagic disease in newborn. Large amts. are toxic.

Effects of Preparation and Storage	Good Sources	NRC Recommended Daily Dietary Allowances
Gradual destruction by oxidation when exposed to high dry temperatures. Stable to heat and usual cooking methods.	Dark green leafy vegetables such as spinach, chard, beet greens, dandelion greens. Deep yellow vegetables and fruits such as carrots, winter squash, sweet potatoes, mangos, cantaloupes, papayas, persimmons, apricots. Broccoli, tomatoes Cream, butter, margarine, whole milk, egg yolk, cheese made with whole milk. Fish liver oils, liver.	Infants, birth to 1 yr. 1500 I.U. Children, 1-3 yrs. 2000 I.U. 3-6 yrs. 2500 I.U. 6-10 yrs. 3500 I.U. 10-12 yrs. 4500 I.U. Teen-agers and adults 5000 I.U. Pregnancy 6000 I.U. Lactation 8000 I.U.
Stable to heat and oxidation.	Sunlight. Fish liver oils. Irradiated foods. Vitamin D milk. Small amounts in egg yolk, liver, butter, cream.	Infants and children, 400 I.U. Adolescents and young adults to age 22 yrs. 400 I.U. Pregnancy and lactation 400 I.U. Other adults No allowances.
Stable to ordinary cooking methods. Destroyed by irradiation, ultraviolet light, iron salts, and rancid fat.	Wheat germ and germ of other cereals. Oils of cottonseed and other seeds. Peanuts, corn, soybeans, nuts, other legumes, whole grain cereals; green leafy vegetables are fair sources.	Infants, birth to 1 yr. 5 I.U. Children, 1-6 yrs. 10 I.U. 6-10 yrs. 15 I.U. 10-14 yrs. 20 I.U. Adolescents, 14-18 yrs. 25 I.U. Men, 18-75 yrs. 30 I.U. Women, 18-75 yrs. 25 I.U. Pregnancy and lactation 30 I.U.
Generally stable to heat, air, moisture. Destroyed by ultraviolet light, alkalies, oxidizing agents.	Alfalfa, cauliflower, cabbage. Soybean oil. Green leafy vegetables. Widely distributed in other foods. Synthesized in intestines.	Not established. Infant, 1 microgram, daily, suggested.

WATER-SOLUBLE VITAMINS (VITAMIN C)

Names	Functions in the Body	Some Symptoms of Deficiency	Effects of Preparation and Stora
Ascorbic Acid	Aids in metabolism of amino acids, absorption of iron, activity of folacin, enzymes in maintaining healthy gums and teeth. Prevents scurvy.	Scurvy. Subacute symptoms. Delayed wound and fracture healing. Hindered bone development and stunted growth. Secondary anemia.	Most unstable vitamin Unstable to heat, air, alkaline, enzymes, copper. Lost by aging, drying, in cooking water. Fairly stable in acid.

WATER-SOLUBLE VITAMINS (B VITAMINS)

Names	Functions in the Body	Some Symptoms of Deficiency	Effects of Preparation and Stora
Thiamine Vitamin B_1	Necessary for metabolism of carbohydrates. Is growth factor. Promotes appetite. Essential for proper function of heart, nerves, and muscles.	Beriberi. Retarded growth. Fatigue, insomnia, poor powers of concentration. Anorexia, constipation. Nervousness, irritability, depression.	Unstable to moist hea and alkali (such as soda). Destroyed by sulfite, and prolonged hea Dissolved in cooking water. Stable to dry heat or in acid media, to atmospheric condi
Riboflavin Vitamin B_2	Is essential component of enzyme systems. Involved in metabolism of carbohydrate, amino acids. Helps to maintain healthy eyes and skin.	Itching, burning eyes. Eyestrain, sensitivity to light, cataract. Cheilosis. Sore, red tongue and mouth. Dermatitis.	Destroyed by alkali. Deteriorates when exposed to sunlight, light. Stable to heat, air, an acid of ordinary cooking methods.

od Sources	NRC Recommended Daily Dietary Allowances
ry little storage—needed on a daily basis. rus fruits, berries, melons, green peppers, dark green leafy vegetables, cabbage, potatoes, guavas, tomatoes, rose hips, and many subtropical and tropical fruits.	In milligrams Infants, 0-1 yr. 35 mg. Children, 1-12 yrs. 40 mg.; 12-14 yrs. 45 mg. Boys and men, 14-18 yrs. 55 mg.; 18-75 yrs. 60 mg. Girls and women, 14-18 yrs. 50 mg.; 18-75 yrs. 55 mg. Pregnancy and lactation, 60 mg.

od Sources	NRC Recommended Daily Dietary Allowances
rms of cereals. gumes, especially soybeans and peanuts. ole grain or enriched cereals and flour. een leafy vegetables. ewers' yeast.	In milligrams Infants, 0-1 yr. 0.2, 0.4, 0.5 mg.; Children, 1-10 yrs. 0.6, 0.7, 0.8, 1.0, 1.1 mg. Boys, 10-12 yrs. 1.3 mg.; 12-14 yrs. 1.4 mg.; 14-18 yrs. 1.5 mg. Men, 18-35 yrs. 1.4 mg.; 35-55 yrs. 1.3 mg.; 55-75 yrs. 1.2 mg. Girls, 10-12 yrs. 1.1 mg.; 12-18 yrs. 1.2 mg. Women, 18-75 yrs. 1.0 mg. Pregnancy 0.1 mg. Lactation 0.5 mg.
k, cheese, eggs. een leafy vegetables. er and meat. ole grain or enriched cereals and flour. ast, dry. gumes, nuts.	In milligrams Infants, 0-2 mo. 0.4 mg.; 2-6 mo. 0.5 mg.; 6 mo.-2 yrs. 0.6 mg.; 2-3 yrs. 0.7 mg. Children, 3-4 yrs. 0.8 mg.; 4-6 yrs. 0.9 mg.; 6-8 yrs. 1.1 mg.; 8-10 yrs. 1.2 mg.; 10-12 yrs. 1.3 mg.; 12-14 yrs. 1.4 mg. Boys and men, 14-18 yrs. 1.5 mg.; 18-22 yrs. 1.6 mg.; 22-75 yrs. 1.7 mg. Girls and women, 14-16 yrs. 1.4 mg.; 16-75 yrs. 1.5 mg. Pregnancy 1.8 mg.; lactation 2.0 mg.

WATER SOLUBLE VITAMINS–Continued

Names	Functions in the Body	Some Symptoms of Deficiency	Effects of Preparation and Storag
Niacin Nicotinic acid Nicotinamide Niacin equivalent: 60 mg. tryptophan forms 1 gm. niacin	Essential component of enzyme systems and in metabolism. Helps to maintain normal function of nervous and digestive systems, and skin. Aids in cell respiration.	Pellagra. Forgetfulness, irritability, depression.	Stable to heat, air, light, alkalies and acids.
Vitamin B_6 Pyridoxine Pyridoxal	Essential in metabolism of polyunsaturated fats, amino acids, carbohydrate. Involved in production of niacin from tryptophan. Increased need during pregnancy, especially toxemias.	Impaired growth, anemia, convulsions in infants. Weakness, depression, sleepiness, anorexia, nausea. Anemia, kidney stones.	Destroyed by ultraviol light and heat. Lost in milling. Stable to strong acids and alkalies.
Vitamin B_{12} Cobalamin	Needed for growth and normal functioning of all body cells and for red cell formation. Involved in metabolism. Beneficial in pernicious anemia.	Pernicious anemia. Other not fully established effects.	Destroyed by heat. Gradually destroyed b strong acids or alkalies and by ligh
Folacin Folic Acid Pteroylglutamic acid (PGA)	Essential for growth, hemoglobin formation, and reproduction. Related to choline synthesis and amino acid metabolism. Connected with function of vitamin B_{12}	Macrocytic anemia. Tropical sprue	Destroyed readily by heat and acid. Deteriorates if expose to sunlight or if stored at room ten perature.

ood Sources	NRC Recommended Daily Dietary Allowances
'eanuts and peanut butter. Brewers' yeast, most dried fruits.)ried peas and beans, some nuts. .iver, lean meats, fish, poultry. Vhole grain or enriched cereals and flour.	In milligram equivalents Infants, 0-2 mo. 5 mg. eq.; 2-6 mo. 7 mg. eq.; 6 mo.-3 yrs. 8 mg. eq.; 3-4 yrs. 9 mg. eq. Children, 4-6 yrs. 11 mg. eq.; 6-8 yrs. 13 mg. eq.; 8-10 yrs. 15 mg. eq. Boys and men, 10-12 yrs. 17 mg. eq.; 12-14 yrs. 18 mg. eq.; 14-18 yrs. 20 mg. eq.; 18-35 yrs. 18 mg. eq.; 35-55 yrs. 17 mg. eq.; 55-75 yrs. 14 mg. eq. Girls and women, 10-14 yrs. 15 mg. eq.; 14-16 yrs. 16 mg. eq.; 16-18 yrs. 15 mg. eq. Pregnancy 15 mg. eq.; lactation 20 mg. eq.
Vheat germ, bran, oatmeal. Vhole grain cereals. Bananas, avocados, some dried fruits. .iver, meat. Soybeans, split peas, peanuts.	In milligrams Infants, 0-2 mo. 0.2 mg.; 2-6 mo. 0.3 mg.; 6 mo.-1 yr. 0.4 mg.; 1-2 yrs. 0.5 mg. Children, 2-3 yrs. 0.6 mg.; 3-4 yrs. 0.7 mg.; 4-6 yrs. 0.9 mg.; 6-8 yrs. 1.0 mg.; 8-10 yrs. 1.2 mg.; 10-12 yrs. 1.4 mg.; 12-14 yrs. 1.6 mg.; 14-18 yrs. (boys) 1.8 mg.; 14-16 yrs. (girls) 1.8 mg.; 16-18 yrs. (girls) 2.0 mg. Adults, 18-75 yrs. 2.0 mg. Pregnancy and lactation 2.5 mg.
Fresh milk, eggs, cheese. Lean meats, liver, kidney. May be small amount of microbial synthesis in intestines.	In micrograms Infants, 0-2 mo. 1.0 mcg.; 2-6 mo. 1.5 mcg.; 6 mo.-2 yrs. 2.0 mcg. Children, 2-3 yrs. 2.5 mcg.; 3-4 yrs. 3 mcg.; 4-8 yrs. 4 mcg. Children and adults, 8-55 yrs. 5 mcg.; 55-75 yrs. 6 mcg. Pregnancy 8 mcg.; lactation 6 mcg.
Green leafy vegetables. Whole grains, legumes, nuts. Yeast, liver, kidney. Small amounts are widely distributed in other foods.	In milligrams Infants, 0-6 mo. 0.05 mg.; 6 mo.-2 yrs. 0.1 mg. Children, 2-8 yrs. 0.2 mg.; 8-10 yrs. 0.3 mg.; 10-18 yrs. 0.4 mg. Men and women, 18-75 yrs. 0.4 mg. Pregnancy 0.8 mg.; lactation 0.5 mg.

Can a Vegetarian Be Healthy?

"What she needs is a good red beefsteak."

"My husband is a construction worker. He does such heavy work that he needs plenty of meat."

"Our son is on the football squad, and the coach orders a thick steak every day."

Such remarks as these are not unusual. You have no doubt heard similar ones. They reflect the widely held belief that meat is necessary to maintain strength and vigor. Many people assume that vegetarians, people who eat no meat, are anemic and weak. Is there a basis for these popular beliefs? Is it possible for a vegetarian to get an adequate diet, to be strong and healthy?

Most people of the world subsist on a largely vegetarian diet, usually from necessity due to scarcity or prohibitive cost of foods of animal origin. Some groups and individuals follow a vegetarian regimen from choice or from hygienic, religious, or philosophical convictions. Is this practice nutritionally sound?

Before considering these questions let's define terms by classifying dietary practices as (1) nonvegetarian—including foods of animal origin as well as plant foods; (2) lacto-ovo-vegetarian—using foods of plant origin plus milk and eggs; and (3) vegetarian—living exclusively upon plant foods with no foods of animal origin, sometimes termed strict or pure vegetarian.

In common usage the term vegetarian may denote a diet without flesh foods but including milk and eggs—technically, lacto-ovo-vegetarian.

Vegetarianism is not new. It is as old as the world itself with the Creator prescribing a diet of fruits, nuts, grains, and "the herb of the field." Following the Flood, plant foods were not immediately available; therefore God told man, "Every moving thing that liveth shall be meat for you." In Leviticus 11 and Deuteronomy 14 distinction is recorded between clean and unclean meats.

In recent years concern over the population explosion and the nutritional needs of developing countries has caused scientists to take a close look at plant foods and vegetarianism.

Protein content or quality has usually been the prime consideration, but other nutrients—minerals and vitamins, particularly iron and calcium, vitamin B_{12}, and possibly riboflavin—and such factors as cholesterol and diseases of animals are also of valid concern.

Protein. Protein needs are influenced by age, size, body structure, stress, and disease but not by physical activity. As Dr. Frederick Stare of Harvard has expressed it, the demand of lumberjacks for plenty of red meat is based on habit and desire, not nutritional need.

By Western Hemisphere standards the nonvegetarian diet has been considered by the majority as indispensable to health. Leading biochemists and nutritionists, however, such as Dr. Henry C. Sherman of Columbia University, Dr. E. V. McCollum of Johns Hopkins University, and others have for years been pointing out the excellence of the lacto-ovo-vegetarian diet.

Adequate protein is essential at all ages; and animal foods including milk, cottage and other cheese, eggs, meat, fish, and poultry provide protein of good quality. Some plant foods, such as cooked soybeans and garbanzos, wheat germ, and food yeast, contain good protein; but the protein of most plant foods is not as complete as that from animal sources or is present in small amounts.

In recent years, however, there has been a shift from emphasis on the protein quality of individual foods to amino acid requirements and supplementation. A complete protein does not necessarily have to come from a single food. It can be from a mixture of two or more incomplete or partially complete proteins that together form the right proportions of essential amino acids. This is called supplementation. In other words, amino acids of one food can combine with those of another to form a complete protein.

Sometimes a "reference protein," with an ideal ratio of essential amino acids for tissue synthesis in the body, is used as a standard. Whole egg may be taken as the standard for the amino acid pattern with a score of 100, and other foods are rated in reference to it. This is termed chemical evaluation.

Animal feeding experiments are another means of evaluating proteins. These sometimes reveal biological values which differ markedly from the chemical evaluation scale. This is because factors other than amino acid balance influence the protein values, such as digestibility, toxic substances found naturally in some plant foods, microorganisms that develop under certain conditions, and heat processing.

Excessive heat treatment over a prolonged period of time may make proteins unavailable. This has been the reason for poor protein evaluations in some studies. Proper heat treatment, on the other hand, may improve protein quality. Some of the legumes are an example. They may contain toxic substances which are inactivated by cooking.

Most plant proteins are low in one or more of the amino acids—lysine, tryptophan, threonine, or methionine. Cereal grains are low in lysine, while legumes are high in lysine but low in methionine in which cereals are adequate. The two combined thus supplement each other and may provide good protein.

To better illustrate supplementation possibilities, the chart below lists some plant foods and the amino acids in which they are adequate and those in which they are limited.

Amino Acids

SOME FOOD SOURCES OF PROTEIN	AMPLE OR EXCESS AMOUNTS OF AMINO ACIDS	LIMITED AMOUNTS
Most cereals and millets	methionine	lysine, threonine
Corn		lysine, threonine, tryptophan
Most legumes	lysine, threonine	methionine, cysteine tryptophan
Soybeans	lysine, threonine	methionine
Sesame and sunflower seeds	methionine, cysteine and tryptophan	lysine
Peanuts		lysine, threonine, methionine
Green peas	lysine	methionine
Green leafy vegetables		methionine
Brazil nuts	methionine	

Through the ages people have practiced amino acid supplementation instinctively. Cereals and legumes, and milk and cereals are commonly used together. For instance in India rice and dhal (a variety of lentils) and in Central America corn and beans are commonly eaten together.

Supplementation may also be achieved by the addition of synthetic amino acids to foods. Cereals may be fortified by the addition of synthetic lysine. Care must be exercised in the use of this method, though, since an excess of an amino acid may be toxic or cause imbalance of other nutrients. Supplementing with foods is usually to be preferred and is cheaper.

Some reports of experimental vegetarian diets have seemed to indicate inadequacy of protein. One must always take into consideration, however, the conditions under which the experiment is conducted, and these vary.

Using white rats, Dr. Cecile Edwards fed a basic diet of cornbread, sweet potatoes, collard greens, and fatback. She added one kind of legume at a time. Results, compared to those with a standard rat ration, were disappointing. Growth responses were limited and different for each legume. Even the addition of skim milk, however, improved growth only in some cases, so results could not be entirely due to amino acid deficiency of the legumes.

"Just because plant foods, when fed alone, do not provide the necessary quota of essential amino acids is no reason to condemn them as protein sources. . . . When a variety of plant foods is used, one food tends to make up for the deficiencies of another," states Corinne H. Robinson in *Fundamentals of Normal Nutrition,* 1968, page 63.

A number of studies in this country and abroad in which legumes have been combined with cereals, nuts, and oil seeds obtained results similar to those in which meat was used. Some animal studies with lacto-ovo-vegetarian diets in meal patterns such as usually eaten at a family table have reported normal growth and satisfactory nitrogen balance.

Dr. Albert Sanchez, as reported in the *Journal of the American Dietetic Association* in 1966, tested the nutritional value of various diets by the rat-growth method. Those which included milk resulted in the best growth rates, and the one which contained vegetable protein entrées with milk and eggs compared favorably with the same diet in which meats replaced the vegetable entrées.

Dr. U. D. Register at Loma Linda University formed three equal groups of students into experimental teams. He fed one group a vegetarian diet, the second group a lacto-ovo-vegetarian diet, and the third group a nonvegetarian diet, each containing sixty grams of protein a day, for seventeen days. All three groups maintained nitrogen balance. In a further study a vegetarian diet at a thirty-five-gram protein level was fed for seventeen days to six young men and women. Four remained in nitrogen balance. The amino acid content of all the diets exceeded the established minimal requirements.

Variety in the use of wholesome foods is the best insurance of securing high quality protein. In the United States there seems to be little concern regarding protein deficiency for adults getting sufficient calories from a varied diet. Children, however, may be protein deficient on a vegetarian program unless careful attention is given to their diets. Proteins must be supplied to small children in a form which their systems are able to utilize. For instance, children might be served cottage cheese instead of cured cheeses. They can be given smooth nut butters rather than whole nuts, and entrées should be made from ground nuts rather than large nut pieces.

Research teams in many countries are earnestly studying economical and locally available plant protein sources and exploring the possibilities of increasing protein values by mutual supplementation.

International agencies such as the World Health Organization, Food and Agriculture Organization, and the United Nations Children's Fund, combine efforts to improve the nutritional status of the world. They provide research grants for the purpose of finding cheap sources of protein in areas where the normal diet is deficient. In general, the plan involves the supplementation of cereal grains, which form the staple food in most developing areas, with other available plant proteins such as legumes, oil seeds, palm kernels, and leaf proteins.

In Central America a suitable, low-cost protein mixture which closely resembles the quality of milk protein has been developed. It consists of cottonseed flour mixed with maize meal, sorghum meal, and torula yeast. This is very acceptable as a thin gruel and is now on the market under the name Incaparina.

In India many plant foods are being studied such as mixtures of peanut flour with Bengal gram or sesame flour. Emphasis has been on locally grown protein-rich plant food combinations for children. A mixture of pulses (legumes similar to lentils) has been prepared. Some experiments compared the regeneration of protein in blood plasma when skim milk, chick-peas, and rice diets were fed. The milk and chick-pea diets were about equivalent, both higher than the rice diet. Both the milk and the chick-pea diets were successful in treating malnutrition.

A soybean and sesame flour mixture is being produced in Indonesia under the name Saridele. In Senegal millet meal and peanut flour mixtures have proved almost equal in value to millet-milk mixtures in treating undernourished children. In Nigeria various plant mixtures with skim milk have been given to the very young or malnourished. Uganda has used a mixture of whole peanuts with skim milk and cottonseed oil for large-scale feeding programs. Other areas around the world are discovering vegetable protein mixtures of locally available foods.

It is evident from the preceding information that a vegetarian diet can be adequate as far as protein is concerned. Comments from well-known nutrition authorities further confirm this.

Drs. Anthony A. Albanese and Louise A. Orto, writing in *Modern Nutrition* by Wohl and Goodhard, 1968, state, "By proper selection and combination of plant proteins it is possible to devise meals which supply the necessary amino acids in satisfactory quantities. The old nutritional belief that diets containing animal proteins are necessarily superior to those composed entirely of vegetable proteins is therefore valid only with qualifications. . . . Much of our thinking in this area will have to be revised."

"Food," The Yearbook of Agriculture, 1959, puts it this way: "We have come to realize that perhaps some of the chemical units that make meat, milk, and eggs superior foods for filling the protein needs of people may be supplied by skillfully combining certain foods from plant sources in special proportions. For that, our knowledge of the chemistry and requirements of amino acids is most useful."

Dr. Philip L. White, secretary of the Council on Foods and Nutrition of the American Medical Association, was asked, "Is it possible for a vegetarian to obtain all the necessary nutrients to maintain good health?" He answered in *Today's Health* of June, 1966: "It is possible, but somewhat difficult. Special care must be taken to include whole grain cereals, legumes, nuts, and nutlike seeds as well as a wide variety of vegetables and fruits. This wide variety is necessary in order for people to be assured of an adequate intake of the more difficult to obtain vitamins, folic acid, and vitamin B_{12}, as well as calcium and iron.

"The lacto-ovo-vegetarian has an easier time, since eggs, milk, and milk products may be consumed. These foods help assure adequate amounts of protein, calcium, and the B vitamins."

To the question, "Can an adequate diet be secured without meat, milk, or eggs?" Dr. Frederick Stare replied, "It is not absolutely necessary that milk and eggs be included in the diet if meat is omitted. An adequate amount of protein can be obtained by using mixed whole grains, legumes, and nuts; but it is far simpler to be sure of adequate protein if milk and eggs are included.

"It is still sometimes stated that vegetable protein is deficient in certain essential amino acids and can never wholly replace animal protein. . . . Not only is protein from animal sources unnecessary, but also it is not even essential that we receive protein as such from any source as long as we consume the essential amino acids in proper quantities together with a utilizable source of nitrogen for biosynthesis of the 'nonessential' ones."

Notice this confirming statement: "While most individual vegetable proteins are relatively deficient in one or more amino acids, the deficiency can frequently be corrected by combining them with other vegetable proteins of complementary amino acid composition."—Nevin S. Scrimshaw, head of the Department of Nutrition and Food Science, Massachusetts Institute of Technology. Given at Western Hemisphere Nutrition Conference, 1965.

Minerals and Vitamins. Most minerals and vitamins are supplied satisfactorily on any good mixed diet. According to present knowledge a well-balanced lacto-ovo-vegetarian regimen is adequate in all respects; but on a pure vegetarian diet the inclusion of ample calcium, iron, vitamin B_{12}, and perhaps even riboflavin requires careful planning.

Figures in food composition tables may give a false sense of security as to calcium and iron content of vegetarian diets. Several factors may interfere with the utilization of calcium and iron by the body. Large amounts of fiber hinder calcium absorption, and the fiber content of vegetarian diets has been reported to be as much as four times higher than the nonvegetarian.

Most green leafy vegetables are good sources of calcium and iron. Some (spinach, beet greens, chard) contain an amount of oxalic acid that may form insoluble salts with calcium and iron, which are then not absorbed by the body. Whole grain cereals and breads are usually included in ample quantities in vegetarian diets. They are excellent sources of nutrients and are a desirable part of the diet. They contain phytic acid, which may form insoluble salts with calcium and iron. (Note page 95.)

Milk is an excellent source of calcium in a form well utilized by the body. The calcium of broccoli, cauliflower, and kale is reported to rank almost with milk in availability, but these are not rich sources.

Vitamin B_{12} is found almost entirely in animal foods, although some studies have reported traces in certain plant foods. It is produced by the action of certain bacteria.

The blood levels of vitamin B_{12} in vegetarians have been found to be low but do not always correlate with any deficiency symptoms. Protein content of the diet seems to be a factor in the development of vitamin B_{12} deficiency symptoms. Studies comparing British, Dutch, and American vegetarians showed that the British had more vitamin B_{12} deficiency symptoms than the others. It was found that the British had a protein intake of seven percent of the total calories, whereas the Dutch had nine percent and the Americans had 10.4 percent. A desirable protein intake is thought to be 10 to 15 percent of the total calories.

Some persons on limited vegetarian diets have been reported with symptoms such as sore mouth, pain and stiffness in the back and legs, numbness of hands and feet, and other nervous manifestations. Injections of vitamin B_{12} and change to a lacto-ovo-vegetarian diet improved their conditions dramatically.

Vitamin B_{12} may be stored in the body for several years, but some vegetarians have in time exhibited a deficiency. Vitamin B_{12} is associtated with pernicious anemia, and injections of the vitamin are effective treatment in most cases.

Vitamin B_{12} is needed in only minute amounts. Including milk and eggs in the diet or fortifying some of the staple foods of vegetable origin with vitamin B_{12} solves the problem for the average individual on a vegetarian diet.

The adult recommended allowances are for calcium, 800 milligrams; iron, 10 milligrams for men and 18 milligrams for women; riboflavin, 1.7 milligrams for men and 1.5 milligrams for women; vitamin B_{12}, 5 micrograms per day.

The following menu, which uses the daily food guide as a pattern, is adjusted for non-vegetarian, lacto-ovo-vegetarian, and vegetarian regimens with calculations of their respective calcium, iron, and riboflavin content using figures from the United States Department of Agriculture Home and Garden Bulletin No. 72. Estimation of vitamin B_{12} content was not attempted, since figures from sources vary widely.

Effort was made to choose generally available plant foods with highest calcium content. You will note that the nonvegetarian and lacto-ovo-vegetarian diets are adequate in calcium and riboflavin while the vegetarian is low and that all three are, according to calculations, adequate in iron for men but not for women. The iron in the vegetarian diet may not be as effectively used as in the lacto-ovo-vegetarian and nonvegetarian diets. Note Comparison of Day's Menu in Calcium, Iron, and Riboflavin on chart on next page.

Cholesterol. The effects of fat intake and serum cholesterol on atherosclerosis have been investigated in short-term and long-range studies. Researchers generally conclude that there is a definite relationship.

Diets of plant foods have tended to lower cholesterol levels in the blood serum. This may be due to lower cholesterol and fat in plant foods, to the amount of polyunsaturated fats they contain, or to the ratio of sugars and starches.

The cholesterol levels of Yemenite Jews who immigrated to Israel, where a diet abundant in animal foods is available, were higher than their brothers in Yemen who fared mainly on a vegetarian diet.

Trappist monks living on a lacto-ovo-vegetarian diet had lower cholesterol levels than Benedictine monks with a diet similar to that of the average American.

Dr. Mervyn Hardinge, while studying at Harvard, conducted a study of vegetarians, lacto-ovo-vegetarians, and nonvegetarians. He measured the cholesterol levels of the three groups in his study. The

COMPARISON OF DAY'S MENU IN CALCIUM, IRON, AND RIBOFLAVIN*

Adult Day's Recommended Allowances: Ca 800 mg; Iron 10-18 mg; Riboflavin 1.5-1.7 mg.

	Non-Vegetarian			Lacto-ovo-Veg.			Vegetarian		
Food Items	**Ca**	**Iron**	**Ribo**	**Ca**	**Iron**	**Ribo**	**Ca**	**Iron**	**Ribo**
1 pint milk	576	0.2	.84	576	0.2	.84			
1 pint soybean milk							95	3.6	.13
3 slices white bread, enriched	48	1.8	.12						
3 slices whole wheat bread				49	1.5	.09	49	1.5	.09
2/3 cup oatmeal	14	0.9	.05	14	0.9	.05	14	0.9	.05
3 oz. roast beef	11	3.2	.19						
2/3 cup baked beans with tomato				118	3.4	.09	118	3.4	.09
1 egg	54	2.3	.28	54	2.3	.28			
12-15 almonds or cashews							38	0.7	.13
1 medium sweet potato	44	1.0	.07	44	1.0	.07	44	1.0	.07
2/3 cup broccoli	88	0.8	.20	88	0.8	.20	88	0.8	.20
2/3 cup coleslaw	35	0.3	.04	35	0.3	.04	35	0.3	.04
1 orange, medium	67	0.3	.06	67	0.3	.06	67	0.3	.06
2/3 cup grapes, raw American type	10	0.3	.02	10	0.3	.02	10	0.3	.02
Total	947	11.1	1.87	1055	11.0	1.74	558	12.8	.88

*Figures from USDA Bulletin No. 8 and Home and Garden Bulletin No. 72.

DIETARY FAT INTAKE AND SERUM CHOLESTEROL LEVELS OF VEGETARIAN AND NONVEGETARIAN GROUPS

Groups	Fat Intake (gm.)	Percent of Calories From Fat	Cholesterol (mg./100 ml.*)
Adults			
Males			
Lacto-ovo-vegetarians	107.6	33.1	243
"Pure" vegetarians	130.2	35.2	206
Nonvegetarians	175.5	43.0	288
Females			
Lacto-ovo-vegetarians	92.2	33.3	269
"Pure" vegetarians	96.9	34.2	206
Nonvegetarians	124.2	41.7	295

*Bloor's method. Results approximately 7.5 percent higher than results by Schoenheimer and Sperry's method.

following table adapted from the *American Journal of Clinical Nutrition,* June, 1962, gives the results:

Dr. Hardinge concluded that serum cholesterol levels of adult vegetarian groups tended to be lower than the adult lacto-ovo-vegetarian and nonvegetarian groups

Dr. L. W. Kinsell observed that when polyunsaturated fats replaced saturated ones in the diet, regardless of the quantity of fat, cholesterol levels decreased. Most vegetable fats are polyunsaturated while animal fats are largely saturated.

Prevalence of Disease Among Animals

Disease among animals is a factor to consider when deciding your choice of diet, since a number of animal diseases have been found to be transmitted to man through food.

Scarcely a year passes without a new disease problem being recognized in the animal kingdom. Approximately ten percent of all farm animals die each year from disease or parasitemia. The livers from approximately fifteen percent of the cattle slaughtered under Federal inspection are condemned as unfit for human consumption, but not all cattle are inspected. A fifth or more of the cattle and swine slaughtered in this country are, according to reports, not subjected to Federal inspection.

Trichinosis is said to be one of the most common parasitic diseases affecting people in the United States, yet little effort is made to inspect pork for trichinosis on the premise that a sufficiently accurate and simple method for detection has not been devised.

Other common diseases to which animals are subject and which may be transmitted to man are tuberculosis, salmonella, brucellosis, and tumors.

In Summary

A lacto-ovo-vegetarian program containing a variety of fruits and vegetables, milk, eggs, ample protein foods, and bread and cereals is an excellent diet, adequate in all the nutrients. The vegetarian diet, to be nutritionally adequate, must be carefully planned and chosen with due regard to amino acid balance, vitamins, especially vitamin B_{12} and riboflavin, and the minerals, particularly calcium and iron.

"Fruits, grains, and vegetables, prepared in a simple way, free from spice and grease of all kinds, make, with milk or cream, the most healthful diet. They impart nourishment to the body, and give a power of endurance and a vigor of intellect that are not produced by a stimulating diet."—Ellen G. White, *Counsels on Health,* page 115.

Food Fad or Fact?

A social worker, visiting a home in her area, found the children hungry and crying. The mother had no food to feed them, but the worker noticed an expensive vitamin-mineral preparation on a kitchen shelf. A door-to-door salesman had persuaded the mother that it could supply her children with the nourishment that their diet lacked. She paid for the tablets with welfare money which could have provided her family with good food for a week or two. The underprivileged mother is not the only one, unfortunately, who is beguiled by the lure of the food quack. She has the company of at least ten million fellow Americans.

A Senate hearing brought out that Americans throw away an estimated billion dollars every year on "misrepresented, unnecessary, or worthless health products and services." Much of it is being spent for food fads. Wallace F. Janssen, writing for the *Journal of the American Dietetic Association,* said, "At the present more 'bunk' is being peddled to the public concerning food than on any other subject."

The dictionary defines a fad as a custom followed for a time with exaggerated zeal, a craze. Fads often contain a germ of truth or are based on twisted scientific facts. Faddists frequently extol the virtues of a particular food. Some such items advocated by them are good food if used sensibly and moderately along with an otherwise adequate diet. But one of the most dangerous facets of food faddism is that some particular food may be recommended as the sole source of nutrients, as a cure-all, or as essential to well-being.

The vitamin-mineral business is one of the most lucrative food fads for their manufacturers. Americans spend millions of dollars annually for the concentrates. The body does need vitamins and minerals; but with all the wonderful fresh foods available in American markets, it should not be necessary to take our nutrients in tablet form.

Without doubt some people are benefited by concentrates, but there are several reasons why their promiscuous use can be dangerous: (1) Vitamin pill users tend to believe that their nutritional needs can be met with a daily tablet, no matter how poor the quality of their diet. (2) The increase of one mineral or vitamin sometimes aggravates the need for others. (3) The theory that if a little is good, more is better does not apply to vitamin-mineral concentrates. Instances have been reported of illness due to overdosage of particular vitamins or minerals. (4) Concentrates lack certain trace elements and no doubt undiscovered vitamins as well. The wisest plan is to eat good, wholesome food and to use mineral and vitamin concentrates with discretion.

Some food fads and fallacies are comparatively harmless; others are dangerous. Mrs. Green's case is typical of those who rely on food fads for a cure of serious illnesses. Mrs. Green was a charming and intelligent woman in her late thirties or early forties. She had been ailing for some time but relying on a "sure-cure" diet. She finally went for treatment to a hospital, and the doctor's examination and the laboratory and X-ray findings revealed that she had waited too long. If she had only consulted a competent physician six months earlier, or even three months, surgical removal of a malignant growth would have been possible. Now there was nothing that medical science could do but try to make her as comfortable as possible. Unfortunately hers is not an isolated case. Seriously ill individuals too frequently follow this fad and that, and seek reliable medical advice too late. Following fads tends to give one a false sense of security.

Equally serious is the effect that food fads, with a resulting inadequate diet, may have upon children. Research studies have shown that the growth years are most important. The harm that is done by severe malnutrition during this period may never be completely erased. Some of the results of poor nutrition which are evident during childhood are poor school performance and difficult behavior patterns, as well as the susceptibility to infections and illness. Following food fads during growth and development may be responsible for one's future poor health and shortened life.

People struggling to lose extra pounds are particularly susceptible to fads. One of the most fertile fields for propagating food fads is the overweight multitude. Every little while a new reducing diet, formula food, gimmick, pill, or slogan such as "calories don't count" makes the rounds. Promises are that pounds will melt away. Sometimes they do temporarily; but usually they return with discouraging suddenness. Often serious malnutrition results from following quack reducing programs no matter how impressive their titles. They are frequently given names which mislead the unwary into believing they are sponsored by reliable sources. One example is the Mayo diet, which has no connection with the Mayo Clinic. The best and most lasting reducing program continues to be a sensible low-calorie diet with moderate exercise; although, as discussed in the chapter "Figure Trimming?" many factors remain to be solved with reference to overweight.

The chronically ill and ailing are understandably susceptible to fads and fallacies. Food fads flourish especially among the thousands of rheumatic patients. An arthritic, suffering intensely and painfully crippled, often grasps naturally at anything which offers a glimmer of hope for relief. Rheumatics frequently experience unexplained remissions of the disease; and if one of these comes when a fad is being followed, it is given credit for a cure. How one wishes there were foods or diets that would alleviate the pain of every rheumatic sufferer! To date no diet cure has been discovered; but an adequate diet, restricted in sugars and calories (especially if there is overweight) and high in vitamins and minerals, is beneficial.

The aged are another group of unfortunate prey for food fads. The quest for the fountain of youth began long before the days of Ponce de León, and none of us is immune to its appeal. Today the search involves millions of Americans and numerous fad diets and devices. Unfortunately most of our older citizens can least afford, either physically or financially, to waste money on fads and fallacies.

It would take a book to discuss all of the food fads. New fads are constantly emerging. They are introduced over the radio and TV, in newspapers, magazines, and books, by a salesman, or by a next-door neighbor.

Food faddists often lose sight of the fact that we need a variety of food. It has become plainer than ever that we do not know all there is to be known about vitamins, minerals, amino acids, carbohydrates, and fats. For example, little attention was paid for years to so-called trace elements, and they were usually dismissed as of little importance in the diet. Now we are recognizing that they are essential to health. Without doubt many more food facts will be discovered in years to come.

Food faddists often have something to sell—a book, a pill, a food, a gimmick. Sometimes their products cannot be purchased in a regular market but must be secured for a high price by mail or at a specialty store or from a door-to-door salesman. They frequently advertise a "precious" product from some out-of-the-way place—a secret formula discovered through long years of research. They tend to cast aspersion on the medical and dietetic professions. They appeal most often to the emotions rather than the intellect.

Examples of food fad advertising methods appeared in a catalog of pills, tablets, food gimmicks, and gadgets. Nearly every one of the approximately one hundred pages had eye-catching illustrations and alluring statements similar to the following:

"New! A fabulous food packed with natural enrichment from a secret formula of Swiss mountain folk!"

"For rich red blood your body needs Superdupe. Pioneered by Health-ee Company and now one of the most talked about of all natural food supplements. It took 100 years of research to produce."

"Are you one of the eight out of ten Americans with calcium deficiency? Take Health-ee Calcee. Get organic minerals from the Gardens of the Sea."

"Insure your body of adequate protein with an easy-to-take, low calorie, ready-to-assimilate, special blend, all-natural, high-quality 93 percent protein pill with *all* the essential amino acids and its own natural digestive enzymes!"

No wonder so many are deluded by fads and fallacies. They are made to sound so much more appealing than good, wholesome, inexpensive food such as bread, milk, cabbage, potatoes, and apples from the market. Food fads sound like an easy step to buoyant health.

The statement made by Dr. Charles Glen King in *Science News-letter* a number of years ago is increasingly true. "Food faddists and nutrition quacks," he said, "are doing great damage to the public by misleading propaganda. Their efforts cause economic loss and wasted expenditure on food fads. . . . What is more serious is the confusion they cause in preventing the public from learning and having confidence in sound nutrition practices." But the claims of faddists are deceptive. It is confusing! How can you avoid being deceived?

Reliable information on nutrition may be secured from the Food and Nutrition Board of the National Research Council, 2101 Constitution Avenue, N.W., Washington, D.C. 20437; The American Medical Association, 535 North Dearborn Street, Chicago, Illinois 60610; and the American Dietetic Association, 620 North Michigan Avenue, Chicago, Illinois 60611. The Food and Drug Administration of the United States Department of Health, Education, and Welfare, and the Human Nutrition Research Division of the United States Department of Agriculture prepare valuable information which is available at small cost from the Superintendent of Documents, United States Government Printing Office, Washington, D.C. 20402.

Great efforts are being made to educate the American public against food and health misinformation. Several Federal agencies are joining in a nationwide study of factors that cause people to be taken in by fads and fallacies, health fakes, and swindles. The Federal Government is not the only organization concerned. Many state and local agencies, the American Medical Association, the American Dietetic Association, and the National Better Business Bureau are among organizations endeavoring to counteract food fads and health fakes. Authentic nutrition books have been published, pamphlets distributed, articles written, and lectures presented—all on the subject of good nutrition without reliance on fad.

Remember food fads are a waste of money, offer a false sense of security, and frequently purchase not good health but poor nutrition. There is no perfect food or one that is a remedy for all ills. The best advice is to eat an adequate diet of fruits and vegetables, milk, protein-rich foods, and whole grain or enriched breads and cereals.

Figure Trimming?

Fifteen million American adults share the problem of overweight and long for an easy way to shed their excess pounds. They are easily beguiled by diet books that make such promises as, "Eat all you want and stay trim!" "Calories don't count!" Many are prey to practically any fad diet that comes along: the banana diet, the grapefruit diet, the cottage cheese diet, the steak diet, the gelatin diet, ad infinitum, as well as sundry liquid formulas.

They discover that by sticking to these diets they can always lose weight, and fast! But to their dismay, pounds bounce back almost immediately as soon as they resume their former fare. So a few months later they are trying another "miracle" diet. As a result their nutrition is often inadequate, and serious complications and organic damage can result.

Statistics tell us that about a fifth of all the adults in the United States are overweight to a degree that can affect their health and longevity. Many teen-agers and children suffer from overweight too. Obesity has become a clinical problem and a real concern to public health workers.

Excess pounds tend not only to shorten life but also to aggravate conditions such as high blood pressure, gall-bladder disorders, bone and joint diseases, hernia, and respiratory difficulties. Overweight increases the incidence of toxemia during pregnancy and delivery problems at childbirth. Latent diabetes may come to the surface under the stress of overweight. Surgery is difficult to perform safely, and the mortality risk is increased 42 percent in the moderately obese and 79 percent in the grossly obese.

"Yes, I'm overweight; but what can I do?" is a question often asked.

"It runs in my family," is the excuse frequently given regarding overweight. And there is certainly some heredity relationship, but just what role heredity plays in human obesity is still unknown. In animals heredity appears to be a factor. For example, certain strains of mice inherit obesity. In humans it has been observed that 10 percent of children of normal parents may become obese. This percentage jumps to from 40 to 50 percent when one parent is overweight and to 80 percent when both parents are overweight; but heredity may not be the only cause. Certainly environment, which includes food habits, cannot be ruled out.

Glands are sometimes made the culprit, and they may be involved in some instances. Endocrine obesity is believed to be rare, however. Body fat of this type usually accumulates in rather peculiar ways, choosing certain sites instead of distributing itself all over the body.

Lack of exercise is known to contribute to overweight, especially in middle age, but it is also a factor in the obesity of the young. In fact, when there is little exercise and an unchanged food intake, pounds accumulate steadily and relentlessly at any age. Physical exercise helps to maintain desirable weight and is necessary during every stage of human life.

It becomes easier to gain weight as one gets older. Activity and body metabolism decrease, but food intake usually remains the same or even increases. As small an amount as 100 excess calories a day can cause a gain of five or more pounds a year. If it were only a three pound gain a year, it would amount to thirty extra pounds in ten years! Remember that the best time to reduce is when you gain the first three pounds.

The most common cause of obesity is overeating and under exercising. Desirable weight is really a matter of balance—balance between the calories eaten and the calories spent. When a society becomes affluent and sedentary, this balance is not maintained. In war, famine, and disaster, obesity is rarely a problem.

Unfortunately for those of us who gain easily, calories do have to be reckoned with. They *do* count. Someone has said that there is no magic way to reduce safely except the magic of pushing away from the table and shaking the head from side to side. Weight control, as many scientific articles state, is a lifetime proposition. If you have a tendency to put on pounds, you will have to watch your diet every day just as you wash your face, brush your teeth, and comb your hair.

Individual caloric requirements vary considerably, however. Some persons gain weight on a moderate food intake, while others eat quantities without appearing to add a pound. When you overstep your needs, whether they are large or small, over a period of time, the excess accumulates as fat.

Why do people overeat? The answer is complex and not all the implications are well-understood.

Feelings of hunger or of satiety determine eating habits in most individuals. Many people seem to have a built-in balancing system which functions unconsciously. Others have to attain this balance by curtailing their food intake or increasing their activity or both.

In the person of normal weight the feelings of satiety are said to be abrupt. When he is satisfied he stops eating, no matter how tempting the food may be. Those who have the tendency to obesity, on the other hand, eat beyond the normal amount even to feeling uncomfortable. Therefore, if you are overweight, you will have to apply the willpower brake to stop eating once you begin.

There may also be differences in the eating patterns of the normal and the overweight. It has been observed that obese persons more often skip meals and then lack the willpower to refrain from over-eating at the next meal. The result—accumulation of excess calories.

Food represents many things to people in addition to nourishment. Food habits are interlaced with an individual's background—his ethnic, religious, or cultural patterns. Severe obesity is often traced to childhood food habits, whereas mild obesity originates later.

There may be psychological reasons for overeating. The case of a young girl whom we shall call Evelyn is an example. She has severe acne. She is not "in" with her group and has no dates. Therefore she raids the refrigerator and the candy box. This decreases her feelings of inadequacy but increases her chubbiness. Thus she has entered upon a vicious cycle. Lynn, on the other hand, is unhappy at home. She fears her father and mother are planning a divorce and feels torn between the two. Her only release from emotional upsets is eating; but she is overweight, and this aggravates her unhappiness. Marian is different.

Good-natured and fat, she is full of fun. She loves to eat, especially syrup-and-cream-decked sundaes and malts. She can consume a whole pizza and still partake of quantities of other foods. Food and fun for her go together, and the richer the food the better. Each girl overeats, but each because of a different problem, psychological or emotional.

Food may be used as a substitute for affection. When this is the case, it is referred to as "psychogenic hunger." While it is more commonly seen in childhood and adolescence, it is not unknown among adults. Psychogenic hunger does not coincide with body hunger and originates mainly from feelings of rejection. According to authorities in the field, psychological factors are often the root causes of obesity.

Certainly not all overweight results from psychological or emotional causes. Sensations of hunger and satiety have been correlated with levels of glucose in the blood. Centers of hunger and satiety are located in the hypothalamus, and they seem to be regulated by stimuli such as from the glucose level. In experiments with animals, destruction of the ventromedial nuclei of the hypothalamus resulted in obesity while destruction of the lateral part resulted in loss of appetite. Possibly this is a mechanism which maintains the balance between hunger and satiety. This might explain cases of obesity without apparent emotional or psychological implications.

Controlling weight is complicated by many problems. Onc may be family attitude. For example, Janice has had a tendency to overeat since she was small. Now nineteen, she is grossly overweight to the dismay of her slim mother. Janice is sensitive to her mother's remarks no matter how well meant. She has tried dieting, which she abhors, and the few pounds she loses quickly return. She feels unhappy and rebellious against her mother. She skips breakfast often and eats small servings at the table, but then she gorges on snacks between meals.

The problem of dealing with obesity is often baffling. Although a low-calorie diet seems logical, it does not always attain the expected results. Food means many things to many people. Food habits, a part of the personality itself, are difficult to change. Skill, time, motivation, and encouragement are needed to break bad food habits and control an insatiable appetite. A big part of the problem is determining the underlying cause in each individual case.

In order for a person to succeed in figure trimming he must have a strong desire to reduce. This is the most important factor. Encouragement by family members, physician, or dietitian, can be a great help. It sometimes works wonders in motivating a person to lose weight.

Experiments in group therapy have produced encouraging results. Some individuals seem to rely more on outside stimuli than on those arising from within themselves, and interaction within a group is dynamic and contagious.

Fad diets, often highly publicized in modern magazines, give the impression that weight loss is a cinch. Often fad diets are nutritionally inadequate and unrealistic and are not satisfactory for a long-term program. Starvation can cause serious complications such as liver damage or heart trouble. A starvation diet never should be attempted without medical supervision.

Formula diets, although planned to be adequate in protein, minerals, and vitamins, do not represent a lasting solution. They become monotonous and lack bulk.

Omission of meals, especially breakfast, is of no advantage. It only results in a ravenous appetite at the following meal and consumption of even more calories.

Salt restriction is not necessary unless salt and water are retained in excess.

Drugs to control appetite may be dangerous. At best they are a crutch. They should never be used indiscriminately, but only under a doctor's orders. Drugs do not correct faulty dietary habits.

Physical exercise is a must. Walking is beneficial at all ages.

When all is said and done, however, the key to losing weight is diet—one which is adequate in all nutrients but moderate in calories. It must be adaptable to each person's food habits and mode of living. If it is not, it will not be followed for long. The diet should be functional and simple and should fill the needs of a lifetime if necessary. Adaptability is the core. Weight control, as has been said, is a lifetime proposition. Weight loss should be slow—usually not more than two pounds a week. Causes for overeating should be corrected first before starting the regimen.

Strenuous reducing programs should not be undertaken except under the direction of a physician. One-thousand-to-fifteen-hundred-calorie diets usually insure moderate weight loss.

The Daily Food Guide is the pattern for the reducing diet. In the milk group skim milk or buttermilk should be used instead of whole.

Ample protein foods low in fat will help to give a feeling of satiety.

Breads and cereals may be used in moderation, while low calorie fruits and vegetables should be used freely. Fruits and vegetables in salads, raw or cooked, add bulk which also can give a feeling of satisfaction. Artificial bulk-producing agents such as methyl cellulose have no merits. Fruit can take the place of high-calorie desserts.

In view of recent reports it would seem wise to use artificial or non-caloric sweeteners sparingly. The National Academy of Sciences recommends that daily consumption not exceed 5 grams. (A twelve-ounce bottle of diet soft drink may contain 1 gram.) Since non-calorie sweeteners are added to many foods on the market this amount is frequently exceeded.

In conclusion, the dream of attaining slimness while eating all the calories you want is an illusion. Calories in foods are there to stay. Overeating above the body's needs inevitably leads to overweight.

The long-term goal of desirable weight, in the absence of organic or metabolic disorders, can be attained when you follow a program of sensible dieting and moderate exercise, relieve the stresses which lead to overeating, and have a powerful desire to lose weight.

MEAL PATTERN

BREAKFAST	**1000 Calories**	**1200 Calories**	**1500 Calories**
Citrus fruit or juice	1 serving	Same	Same
Fruit (see list)	1 serving	Same	Same
Protein food	1 serving	Same	Same
Whole wheat toast or cereal	1 serving	Same	Same
Fat	None	½ serving	1 serving
LUNCHEON OR SUPPER			
Protein food	1 serving	Same	Same
Vegetable—List B (or bread)	1 serving	Same	Same
Fruit (see list)	1 serving	2 servings	2 servings
Bread (or carbohydrate)	1 serving	Same	Same
Fat	1 serving	Same	3 servings
Skim milk or buttermilk	1 cup	Same	Same
DINNER			
Bouillon	1 cup	Same	Same
Protein food	2 servings	Same	Same
Vegetable—List A	As desired	Same	Same
Vegetable—List B	1 serving	Same	Same

Bread (or carbohydrate)	1 serving (if not at lunch)	1 serving	1½ servings
Fruit (see list)	1 serving (if not at breakfast)	Same	3 servings
Fat	None	1½ servings	2 servings
Skim milk or buttermilk	1 cup	Same	Same

SUGGESTED MENUS

1000 Calories

BREAKFAST

Grapefruit—½
Fresh strawberries—½ cup
Poached egg on whole wheat toast
Postum with skimmed milk

LUNCHEON OR SUPPER

Sandwich:
White Chik, soyameat — 1 slice
Lettuce Leaf
Whole wheat bread—2 slices
Butter—1 pat
Mayonnaise—½ tbsp.
Fresh peach—1 medium
Skimmed milk

DINNER

Vegetable bouillon
†Spanish Proteena balls
Cauliflower—½ cup
Mixed greens—½ cup
Lemon juice (for greens)
Carrot, celery, bell pepper sticks
Skim milk or buttermilk

1200 Calories

BREAKFAST

Grapefruit—½
Fresh strawberries—½ cup
Poached egg on whole wheat toast
Margarine—½ pat
Postum with skimmed milk

LUNCHEON OR SUPPER

Sandwich:
White Chik—1 slice
Sliced tomato and lettuce
Whole wheat or rye bread—2 slices
Margarine—1 pat
Mayonnaise—1 tbsp.
Fresh peach—2 medium
Skimmed milk

DINNER

Bouillon—1 cup
†Spanish Proteena balls
Mashed Potatoes—½ cup (with skim milk only)
Margarine—½ pat
Mixed greens—½ cup
Lemon juice (for greens)
Carrot, celery, bell pepper sticks
Skim milk or buttermilk

1500 Calories

BREAKFAST

Grapefruit—½
Fresh strawberries—½ cup
Poached egg on whole wheat toast
Margarine—1 pat
Postum with skimmed milk

LUNCHEON OR SUPPER

Sandwich:
White Chik—1 slice
Sliced tomato and lettuce
Whole wheat or rye bread—2 slices
Margarine—2 pats
Mayonnaise—1½ tbsp.
Fresh peach—2 medium
Skimmed milk

DINNER

Bouillon—1 cup
†Spanish Proteena balls
Baked potato (⅓ lb. size)
Margarine—2 pats
Mixed greens—½ cup
Lemon juice (for greens)
Carrot, celery, bell pepper sticks
Dates—6; or dried figs, 3 small; or sponge cake (1/12 of 8 in. dia. cake); or 1 plain cookie (3 in. dia.)

---

†Recipe for this dish can be found in the companion cookbook series to this volume, *Vegetarian Cookery.*

"A" VEGETABLES
as desired raw,
½ to 1 cup cooked, daily.

Asparagus
Broccoli
Brussels sprouts
Cabbage
Cauliflower
Celery
Cucumbers
Eggplant
"Greens"
Lettuce
Mushrooms
Okra
Peppers, green
Radishes
Sauerkraut
String beans
Summer squash
Tomatoes
Water cress

"B" VEGETABLES
½ cup daily

Beets
Carrots
Onions
Peas, green
Pumpkin
Rutabagas
Squash, winter
Turnips

FRUIT LIST (fresh, canned water pack, or frozen without sugar. May be prepared with non-calorie sweetener.

Apple	1 small
Applesauce	½ cup
Apricots, fresh	2 medium
Apricots, dried	4 halves
Banana	½ small
Berries	1 cup
Cantaloupe	¼ medium
Cherries	10 large
Dates	2
Figs, fresh	2 large
Figs, dried	1 small
Grapefruit	½ small
Grapes	12
Grape juice	½ cup
Honeydew melon	⅛ medium
Orange	1 small
Orange juice	½ cup
Peach	1 medium
Pear	1 small
Pineapple	½ cup
Pineapple juice	⅓ cup
Plums	2 medium
Prunes, dried	2
Raisins	2 tablespoons
Tangerine	1 large
Tomato juice	1 cup
Watermelon	1 cup balls or ½ slice, 1 in. thick

BREAD (OR CARBOHYDRATE) LIST

Bread	1 slice
Cereals, cooked	½ cup
Cereals, dry	¾ cup
Corn	⅓ cup
Potatoes, white,	
baked or boiled,	1 medium
or mashed	½ cup
Potatoes, sweet, yam	¼ cup
Rice or grits, cooked	½ cup
Spaghetti, noodles	½ cup

PROTEIN FOOD LIST

Cheese: Swiss, jack,	1 slice
Cheese, cottage	¼ cup
Egg	1
Vegetable steaks (prepare with 1 teasp. fat)	1
Vegeburger (prepare with 1 teasp. fat)	¼ cup
Soy beans	¼ cup
Soy cheese (tofu)	¼ cup
1 ounce lean meat:	1 thin slice, 4 inches square
Peanut butter (subtract 2 teasp. fat)	2 tbsp.
Legumes	
Garbanzos	
Great northern	
Lima beans	
Lentils	
Split peas	
(subtract half of serving from bread or carbohydrate list)	
Soyameat	
Canned—Fried chicken style, diced or sliced	1/6 can—
Beef style	2 oz.
Frozen—	
White Chik	1 slice—1 oz.
Prime, sliced	1 slice—1 oz
Wham	1 slice—1½ oz.
Dark nutmeat (Proteena)	1 slice—1½ oz.

Vegetable steaks and Vegeburger are canned vegetable protein foods.

FAT LIST

Margarine or butter	1 pat
Mayonnaise	½ tbsp.
French dressing	1 scant tbsp.
Cream (half and half)	2½ tbsp.
Cream, heavy	1 tbsp.
Cream cheese	1 tbsp.
Avocado	¼—10 oz.
Olives	5 medium
Sour cream	2 tbsp.
Oil	1 tsp.

ZERO SALAD DRESSING

½ cup tomato juice
2 tbsp. lemon juice
Salt
1 tbsp. finely chopped onion
Chopped parsley or green pepper may be added, if desired.
Combine ingredients in a jar with tightly fitted top; shake well.

YOU MAY USE AS DESIRED:

Bouillon, clear, fat-free
Broth, clear, fat-free
Coffee substitutes
Flavorings, unsweetened
Gelatin, unflavored or artificially sweetened
Dzerta gelatin
Dill pickles
Salt
Seasoned salt

DO NOT USE

Sugar
Honey
Jam and jelly
Marmalade
Syrups
Pies, pastries
Cakes
Cookies
Condensed milk
Soft drinks
Beer, wine, or other alcoholic beverages
Fried, creamed, or scalloped foods
Candy-coated gum
Candy

WEIGHT IN POUNDS ACCORDING TO FRAME

(in indoor clothing)

	HEIGHT (with shoes on, 1-inch heels) Feet	Inches	SMALL FRAME	MEDIUM FRAME	LARGE FRAME
	5	2	112-120	118-129	126-141
DESIRABLE	5	3	115-123	121-133	129-144
	5	4	118-126	124-136	132-148
WEIGHTS	5	5	121-129	127-139	135-152
	5	6	124-133	130-143	138-156
FOR MEN	5	7	128-137	134-147	142-161
	5	8	132-141	138-152	147-166
of ages 25	5	9	136-145	142-156	151-170
	5	10	140-150	146-160	155-174
and over	5	11	144-154	150-165	159-179
	6	0	148-158	154-170	164-184
	6	1	152-162	158-175	168-189
	6	2	156-167	162-180	173-194
	6	3	160-171	167-185	178-199
	6	4	164-175	172-190	182-204

	HEIGHT (with shoes on, 2-inch heels) Feet	Inches	SMALL FRAME	MEDIUM FRAME	LARGE FRAME
	4	10	92- 98	96-107	104-119
	4	11	94-101	98-110	106-122
DESIRABLE	5	0	96-104	101-113	109-125
	5	1	99-107	104-116	112-128
WEIGHTS	5	2	102-110	107-119	115-131
	5	3	105-113	110-122	118-134
FOR WOMEN	5	4	108-116	113-126	121-138
	5	5	111-119	116-130	125-142
of ages 25	5	6	114-123	120-135	129-146
	5	7	118-127	124-139	133-150
and over	5	8	122-131	128-143	137-154
	5	9	126-135	132-147	141-158
	5	10	130-140	136-151	145-163
	5	11	134-144	140-155	149-168
	6	0	138-148	144-159	153-173

For girls between 18 and 25, subtract 1 pound for each year under 25.

You and Your Heart

The heart starts its rhythmic pulse sometime before birth and continues night and day, year in year out, without any human prompting. Its constant rhythmic beat distributes the blood throughout the body to nourish every cell, tissue, and organ with oxygen and valuable nutrients and to carry away carbon dioxide and waste materials. Blood is pumped out, blood is pumped in, and the heart keeps the blood from becoming stagnant. It is a dynamic, nonstop function throughout life.

"The clock of life is wound but once," the poem goes, "and no man has the power to tell just when the hands will stop." But recent research has shown that heart attacks can be avoided and death from heart disease delayed by observing certain principles. To preserve the health of your heart it matters how you work, how you live, how you eat, and how you relate yourself to the stresses of life.

Today many research teams are exploring factors related to the heart. Whole populations and smaller groups are being studied through surveys and other research techniques to see how the way of living, the diet, and other components are correlated to the incidence of coronary heart disease. Men are more prone to heart disease than women. Women of child-bearing age seldom suffer from heart disease. But after menopause incidence for women is similar to that for men. Dr. Ancel Keys of the University of Minnesota has headed a program which began in Yugoslavia in 1959 and has involved ten thousand men in fourteen areas abroad in addition to two thousand in the United States. Comparison of the death rates with the modes of living in various countries has been made by research teams.

The study of the heart and agents affecting it is not simple. Reports are made on groups, groups are composed of individuals, and each individual is unique and reacts individually.

If there is no record of heart attacks, strokes, or diabetes in your family; if your diet is adequate but low in fat, your exercise ample and regular, your way of life calm and happy without undue stress; if you are not overweight and do not smoke and drink; and, particularly but not necessarily, if you are a woman under fifty—your cholesterol should be low and your chance of a heart attack minimal.

Atherosclerosis has come to the limelight as the number one enemy of the heart. Over half of the deaths in America—more than half a million a year—are attributed to cardiovascular disease, much of it due to atherosclerosis. Coronary artery disease, hypertension, and strokes claim the most victims.

In atherosclerosis, plaques of cholesterol and other materials form in the arteries that feed the heart, in the aorta, and in the cerebral arteries. The blood cannot circulate freely, and blood clots may form and produce a heart attack or a stroke. Can heart disease statistics be changed? Is atherosclerosis preventable? Can it be reversed once it has begun?

Although the results from animal experimentation cannot be applied directly to man, some possible assumptions may be based on the findings of these studies. Two answers have been obtained in working with animals: (1) Atherosclerosis is preventable. (2) The process can be reversed if detected in time.

Reducing serum cholesterol or reversing atherosclerosis is much more difficult than preventing it, however. The proper habits of living and eating should be instituted in childhood.

The American Heart Association has listed risk factors that predispose a person to coronary heart disease. They are high levels of cholesterol or other fatty substances in the blood, overweight, high blood pressure, lack of exercise, smoking, diabetes, and family history of heart attacks in middle age.

To eliminate some of the risk factors and to help change heart disease statistics there are ways to guard your heart. A pamphlet published in 1966 by the Association suggests six: (1) Reduce saturated fats and cholesterol in the diet. (2) Count your calories and avoid excess weight. (3) Control high blood pressure. (4) Don't smoke. (5) Exercise regularly. (6) Have regular medical checkups.

Diet

The quality of diet is a major factor in preventing heart disease. In a discussion of diet and heart disease at the American Dietetic Association convention in 1968, the chairman of the Committee on Nutrition of the American Heart Association, Dr. Robert E. Hodges, recommended some dietary principles to follow: (1) Limit the foods containing cholesterol. (2) Substitute polyunsaturated fats for the saturated fats on a two-to-one basis. (3) Limit total fat in the diet to less than 40 percent of the calories (some medical scientists favor not more than 30 percent). (4) Use more complex carbohydrates, such as cereals and grains, rather than sugar. (5) Avoid or correct obesity. Dr. Hodges stated in answer to a question that excessive use of coffee may contribute to coronary heart disease.

Monkeys are suitable experimental animals because they resemble man in many ways and are prone to atherosclerosis. In a model experiment for one hundred and five weeks, Rhesus monkeys were fed a "typical" American diet high in saturated fats, cholesterol, and calories. Another group was fed a "prudent" diet low in these factors. In measuring blood lipids and arterial wall plaques, 75 percent of the monkeys on the "typical" diet showed fatty streaks and plaques compared with fifteen percent of the ones on the "prudent" diet. Higher cholesterol levels were found in the monkeys on the "typical" diet.

The National Diet-Heart Study was carefully planned and conducted to find out if coronary heart disease could be decreased or prevented in middle-aged American men by altering the amount and type of fat and the amount of cholesterol in the diet.

Following small "feasibility" studies with at least 250 subjects each, six principal investigators in different regions of the United States began the project in August, 1962. The participants were (1) free-living men 45 to 54 years of age and (2) long-term residents of mental institutions. These were double-blind studies in which neither the participants nor the evaluating personnel knew who was on a special fat-modified diet.

The fat was 30 and 40 percent of the total calories, the saturated fats and cholesterol were decreased, and polyunsaturated fats increased.

The polyunsaturated to saturated fat (P/S) ratio in the diets were 1.5 and 2.0. The control diet with a P/S ratio of 0.4, was similar to the usual American diet. In the final report it was stated, "Extensive evidence implicates diet as a key factor in the etiology of atherosclerosis and suggests that the disease can be prevented by changes in diet, particularly by lowering serum cholesterol level."

In a five-year follow-up study in Norway, 412 men thirty to sixty-seven years of age who had experienced and survived heart attacks, all with high serum cholesterol levels, were placed in two groups. One group was placed on a restricted diet with instruction and the other with no diet or instruction. The first group's serum cholesterol and number of recurring heart attacks were significantly reduced.

Cholesterol

Cholesterol is a normal constituent of serum and body tissues. It is a necessary substance although not all of its specific functions are well understood. Cholesterol makes important contributions to the body. It is broken down to bile salts which emulsify fats and fat soluble vitamins. It is the basis of some hormones. A form of cholesterol is transformed into vitamin D.

Part of the cholesterol in your body comes from the foods you eat. The largest percentage is formed in your body cells. Even the arterial walls fabricate some. Foods of animal origin contain cholesterol, whereas plant foods are devoid of it.

In the Framingham, Massachusetts, study sponsored by the National Heart Institute, more than five thousand adults were closely followed and checked and the level of cholesterol in the blood was correlated with the development of coronary artery disease. Other studies have indicated a definite relationship between diet and cholesterol levels.

Dr. Jeremiah Stamler believes decreased cholesterol and saturated fats in the diet are factors of crucial importance.

Convincing evidence indicates that serum cholesterol levels are definitely related to the development of cardiovascular disease. In 1961 eight years of observation were reported on men with serum cholesterol levels below 200 mg. percent. It was found that this group developed heart disease at a rate less than half that of the total population. Observation simultaneously on a group with cholesterol levels of 260 mg. percent or above showed a heart disease incidence of twice that of the average, or four times that of the first group.

In one study serum cholesterol was lowered by cutting down on dietary cholesterol and saturated and total fat. The same effect was produced by substituting polyunsaturated fats for at least part of the saturated fats. The serum cholesterol level in middle age was particularly related to heart disease. With high serum cholesterol levels there were three to four times as many heart attacks.

In the April, 1968, *American Journal of Clinical Nutrition* a study on dietary prevention of heart disease was reported. It involved a total of 581 people from thirty to sixty-nine years of age. The incidence of heart disease was significantly lowered with a cholesterol-lowering diet.

Fat

Observations of man and animals indicate that the blood lipid level may rise or fall according to the kind and amount of fat in the diet.

The effect of animal versus vegetable fat, polyunsaturated versus saturated and their ratios in the diet, the essential versus the nonessential fatty acids have all been discussed in numerous research papers. Many experiments in relation to the changes in serum cholesterol and fat levels have been conducted. Still the mechanism that brings about these changes is unknown. In general polyunsaturated fats seem to result in the lowering of cholesterol in the blood.

The use of polyunsaturated fats has been found to increase the requirements for vitamin E. Fortunately vegetable oils, high in polyunsaturates, are fairly high in vitamin E. In one study older men on a diet high in unsaturated fats showed no deficiency of vitamin E.

Dr. D. M. Hegsted has observed that in general the countries which have a low fat intake also have a low incidence of heart disease. Other changes that accompany a low-fat diet such as a low intake of animal protein, low calcium intake, and high fiber intake may also have a bearing. While further study is needed, he stated that cholesterol level, fat intake, and kind of fat are definite determinants.

The percentage of fat in the diet in relation to death rate has been compared in different countries of the world. For instance Americans, Canadians, Britons, Finns, Australians, and New Zealanders have high percentages of fat in their diets, around 40 percent for Americans, and a correspondingly high death rate from coronary heart disease.

Other nationalities such as the Japanese, Bantus, Italians, and

Chinese have low percentages of fat in the diet, around 10 percent in Japan, and have a low death rate from coronary heart disease.

In parts of Asia and Africa where the people eat a largely vegetarian diet, low in foods of animal origin, calories, fat, and cholesterol, they have a correspondingly low serum cholesterol level throughout their lives. Atherosclerosis and coronary heart disease are rare. On the other hand, tribes using large amounts of meat and milk have been reported to have high serum cholesterol and atherosclerosis.

The Anti-coronary Club in New York City included men from forty to fifty years of age who followed an experimental or "prudent" diet program which included a low fat regimen. Unsaturated fats were used in preference to saturated ones. In four years those following this program showed lower cholesterol levels and the incidence of coronary heart disease had decreased significantly as compared with the general public.

To repeat, a "prudent" diet is one high in polyunsaturated fats and low in calories, cholesterol, and saturated fats, which are generally of animal origin. But coconut oil, chocolate, and hydrogenated cooking fats are also saturated. Olive oil and olives contain a large amount of monounsaturated fats. Liquid vegetable oils and the fats of nuts and cereals are high in polyunsaturated fats.

Carbohydrates and Other Factors

Dr. John Yudkin of the Department of Nutrition at the University of London believes that sugar rather than saturated fat may be responsible for heart disease. He states that a person who consumes four ounces of sugar a day has five times the chance of a heart attack of one who uses only two ounces. He points out that world sugar consumption has more than doubled in the last twenty-five years.

Dr. Ancel Keys contends that if the sugar in the American diet were replaced by fruits, vegetables, and legumes, the serum cholesterol values of the population would be lowered.

Sugar in the diet tends to produce higher cholesterol levels than starch. According to some investigators an abundance of sugar can be as deleterious as high saturated fat intake.

Yemenites living in Israel, where one-fourth to one-third of the carbohydrate is sugar, had higher cholesterol levels than the Yemenites living in their own country where the diet contained more starch.

Other carbohydrates such as cellulose, pectins, and agar which the human body cannot digest have been studied. These substances increase the bulk in the diet. Cellulose had no effect on blood lipids. Large quantities of pectin lowered serum cholesterol. It would be necessary for people to consume more than a normal amount of pectin to observe an effect. Vegetarians subsist on a diet high in cellulose and usually have lower cholesterol. But there may be other more crucial factors associated with lowering cholesterol in vegetarian diets.

In animals excess calories have been found to produce atherosclerosis. Some researchers have reported similar findings with people. In the Framingham study the ten-year incidence of coronary heart disease in both men and women was lower in those with below normal weight and rose as weight increased.

Some minerals and vitamins have appeared in isolated studies to have some effect, but much more research is needed. Sodium may be restricted in some kinds of cardiovascular disease and in some types of high blood pressure. Niacin has a cholesterol-lowering effect, but there are side reactions in some patients who are given niacin therapy. Until more is known about its possible toxic effects, niacin will not be used freely for serum-cholesterol lowering. Ascorbic acid is said to lower cholesterol and may be safely and freely used.

Conclusions

Regardless of your condition of heart health or heart disease, you will benefit by following these basic principles:

- Eat an adequate diet.
- Maintain normal weight.
- Consume no more than moderate or low amounts of fats—25 to 30 percent of the calories.
- Replace most of the saturated fats with polyunsaturated.
- Use a low-cholesterol diet.
- Choose foods high in minerals and vitamins, especially ascorbic acid.
- Substitute starchy foods for sugar, and use less sweets.
- Take regular exercise.
- Do not smoke or drink alcoholic beverages.
- Avoid emotional stress. Stop worrying.
- Retain a positive outlook on life.

When the Doctor Says, "Restrict Sodium"

"Your husband will have to follow a careful program when he goes home, and it will be necessary for him to continue to restrict sodium in his diet for some time, perhaps for the rest of his life," a physician told a wife as she prepared to take her husband home from the hospital. She knew that restricted sodium meant, among other things, little or no salt. But she felt determined to prepare attractive and delicious meals for her husband, despite the no-salt restriction, and to serve them to him in an atmosphere not suggestive of illness or special diets. Her project developed into such an interesting one that she eventually published a popularly written low-sodium cookbook.

If a sodium-restricted diet is prescribed for you or if you must prepare a sodium-restricted diet for a member of your family, do not be unduly alarmed. It is possible to fit the diet into the family menu and make it attractive and appetizing.

Sodium is a mineral normally found in the body. It is essential to life. Animals seem instinctively to realize that they need sodium, and in the wild they have been known to travel long distances to reach salt licks.

The average healthy person consumes three to seven grams of sodium a day and normally excretes 90 percent of it, mostly through the kidneys. Among other functions of sodium is its assisting in the movement of fluid in and out of the tissues and cells of the body.

In certain illnesses sodium is not excreted normally and accumulates, causing water to be held in the tissues. The result is edema (swelling). In these circumstances and for some other conditions, sodium-restricted diets are prescribed.

Sodium may be restricted to only one fourth gram (250 milligrams) a day; or it may be limited to 500 milligrams, 800 milligrams, or 1,000 milligrams. When it is only mildly restricted, the diet may contain 1,500 to 2,000 milligrams (1½ to 2 grams). Sometimes sodium-restricted diets are incorrectly termed salt-free, salt-poor, low-salt, salt-deficient.

The most common source of sodium is salt (chemically known as sodium chloride) which is almost half sodium. You may be surprised to learn that water and most foods, even though they do not taste salty, naturally contain sodium in varying amounts. The sodium content in water varies in different areas. Where it is high, it is sometimes necessary to purchase bottled distilled water to be used in cooking and drinking.

In addition to the natural sodium which is part of food, and the extra salt you add, there are other compounds of sodium in many commercially prepared foods. Sodium propionate, sodium acetate, sodium sulfate, sodium citrate, sodium cyclamate are a few of those appearing on labels.

Regular canned foods, bakery products, and other commercial foods, because they contain salt or sodium in some other form, cannot be a part of sodium-restricted diets. Sodium benzoate is a common preservative added to margarine and some other foods. Accént is a trade name for monosodium glutamate. Baking soda and baking powders contain sodium; so do carbonated beverages and many other items. Sodium compounds are rather frequently listed in fine print; so all labels must be very carefully read. This is essential.

Salt substitutes may be used when they are authorized by your doctor. He will determine which ones, if any, you may use.

Your sodium-restricted diet follows, as far as possible, the normal diet pattern of the Daily Food Guide. In general animal foods such as milk have a relatively high sodium content and can be used only in measured amounts. Sometimes a specially processed low-sodium milk is prescribed. Most plant foods are low in sodium. Cereals and fruits can be used freely, fresh or cooked, without added sodium in the form of salt, baking powder, or soda. Vegetables vary in sodium content, but most of them contain only small amounts and so can be used freely. Legumes such as beans, peas, and lentils are low in sodium content and add needed protein. Use them often unless troubled with flatulence.

The sodium-restricted diet can become very distasteful unless care is taken in its preparation. Cooking attractive and appetizing meals without salt is a challenge to the best cook, but it can be done. The secret is planning colorful menus and seasoning with herbs, seeds and nuts, mild spices, and tart foods. You will need to put into practice good cookery principles, plan pleasing color combinations, and use simple garnishes.

Just as an artist chooses and mixes colors, you may combine seasonings to produce meals that are works of art. When seasonings are added with a light touch, a subtle tantalizing flavor is the result. But beware of a heavy hand. Too much seasoning, like too many cooks, can spoil the broth!

One suggestion that has been a help to some is to set aside a shelf for seasonings that are allowed on the sodium-restricted diet. It makes for greater convenience in food preparation. Plan for the whole family to eat the same food in general. The other members of the family will only need to add salt. They, of course, will not need salt-free bread, butter, and dressings but may use the regular ones. They will also use some other foods not on the sodium-restricted diet. On the following page is a list of low-sodium seasoning aids.

Herbs may be used fresh or dried. The amount of herb will vary, since some herbs are strong and others are mild in flavor. Three to four times as much fresh as dried herb may be used. It may be cut, minced, or crushed.

One or several herbs may be placed in a cloth bag similar to a tea bag. The herb bag may be left in food from a few minutes to overnight. Sometimes an herb bag may be left in food all during the cooking, or it may be added during the last few minutes of cooking and removed before serving.

Fine herbs, or Fines Herbes, is a combination of several herbs. The French variety contains basil, chervil, marjoram, thyme, rosemary, and tarragon. Other combinations are basil, chives, and parsley; or basil, marjoram, thyme, and rosemary. Curry is a combination of spices.

Low-sodium Seasoning Aids

Flavorings	Herbs	Seeds and Nuts	Mild Spices	Miscellaneous
Almond extract	Anise	Anise seed	Allspice	Cocoa†
Lemon extract	Basil	Caraway	Cinnamon	Coconut (no added salt)
Maple extract	Bay leaf	Cardamom	Curry powder	Cranberries
Mint	Caraway	Cumin	Paprika	Dietetic catsup‡
Orange extract	Chives	Dill	Poultry seasoning	Lemon juice
Peppermint	Dill	Juniper	Saffron	Lemon rind
Vanilla extract	Fennel	Nuts	Turmeric	Lime juice
Walnut extract	Fine herbs	Poppy seed		Mushrooms
	Garlic*	Sesame seed		Orange juice
	Marjoram			Orange peel
	Mint			Pimiento
	Onion*			Saccharin
	Oregano			Tomato
	Parsley			
	Purslane			
	Rosemary			
	Sage			
	Savory			
	Sorrel			
	Tarragon			
	Thyme			

*Avoid garlic or onion salt. May use powder.
†Do not use Dutch process or instant mix.
‡With lemon juice, no salt.

Other Cooking Aids

Cream of tartar, plain gelatin, honey, Postum, sodium-free baking powder, white sugar, yeast.

Vegetables, protein dishes, and soups are probably the most difficult to make appetizing without salt. Actually vegetables cooked without salt retain a sweet fresh flavor that is lost in salt cookery. Cook the vegetables in a minimum of water (or in a pressure cooker) a minimum length of time.

Possible seasoning combinations for vegetables are legion. Similar seasonings may be used in protein dishes and soups. Experiment and you will discover many delightful combinations. Try, for four servings, ½ teaspoon dill and ¼ teaspoon rosemary; ¼ teaspoon caraway seed and ¼ teaspoon basil; 2 teaspoons chopped parsley and ¼ teaspoon tarragon; ⅛ teaspoon curry powder and ⅛ teaspoon oregano.

Vegetables which are relatively high in sodium and usually must be omitted from sodium-restricted diets are celery, carrots, turnips, and beets, beet greens and other greens. But there are other colorful and flavorful foods which are low in sodium and may be used, tomatoes and cranberries, for instance. Cranberries are colorful and have a pleasing tang.

Lemons and tomatoes are invaluable when cooking without salt. Lemon may be used to add flavor to everything from soup to dessert. A sprinkle of lemon juice on a vegetable can make you forget that it lacks salt. Fresh or salt-free canned tomatoes and tomato juice may be used alone or with herbs as seasoning for vegetables, protein dishes, soups, salad dressings, sauces, and salads.

Getting a variety of proteins into your sodium-restricted diet may cause problems. There are several approximate protein equivalents to one ounce of meat, some of them higher in calories and most of them much lower in sodium content. Here are several: one-fourth cup unsalted cottage cheese; 1 egg; 1 ounce low-sodium dietetic cheese; 2 tablespoons unsalted peanut butter; ½ cup cooked dry beans, black-eyed peas, split peas, garbanzos, lentils; ⅓ cup cooked soybeans; one ounce wheat germ; one (2-ounce salt-free) gluten cutlet; one ounce sunflower seeds; 1½ ounces walnuts, peanuts, brazil nuts, or almonds. The nuts should be chewed thoroughly or preferably ground and combined with some other food, if they are to be utilized by the body.

Favorite recipes may often be used by omitting salt and other sodium-containing substances. Sodium-free baking powder may be substituted for the regular, if approved by your doctor. You may replace 1 teaspoon of regular baking powder with 1½ teaspoons of sodium-free baking powder which may be purchased in some markets. A pharmacist can make it up from the formula given in American Heart Association booklets. Yeast can be used, and there are many possibilities in baking with it.

Restricted sodium diets are prescribed individually and will vary in amount of sodium. The American Heart Association offers excellent booklets for various levels of sodium restriction. These may be secured through your physician or from the heart association.

Preparing delicious meals without salt is a challenge, but can be done by careful planning and by delicate seasoning with herbs, seeds, nuts, mild spices, and colorful and tart vegetables and fruits.

Fewer Cavities: Dentifrice or Diet?

"We changed toothpaste, and now Freddie has fewer cavities," was a recurrent theme of a television commercial. The theme was apparently designed to appeal to parents; but it probably reached a much wider audience, since nearly everyone has dental problems.

The American Dental Association estimates that there are one billion unfilled cavities in the United States. Ninety-seven percent of the American people have some form of dental disorder and twenty-six million are minus all of their teeth.

Caries (cavities) and other dental diseases are nothing new. While they seem to follow civilization and to be more prevalent and severe in the modern era, they have plagued mankind for thousands of years. Sumerians living before 3,500 B.C. suffered from caries according to archaeological findings. Cavities are even apparent in the fossils of Java man and the Neanderthal man.

Various remedies have been tried throughout the centuries. Relying on a dentifrice is not a modern innovation. More than 4,000 years ago powdered bones of small animals served as tooth powder, and a mouthwash was being used by some Chinese. In Europe, centuries later, bad breath as well as cavities must have been a problem—it was customary to rinse the mouth with wine after meals and sometimes with perfume.

Today dental disease is worldwide. Except in some primitive areas it is the most prevalent of all diseases. Some primitive peoples who never heard of a toothbrush, much less of toothpaste or mouthwash, have been found to have few cavities. Others suffer bad decay. What makes healthy teeth? What causes dental decay? Wrong dentifrice? Poor diet? Or are there other influences?

Scientists have been searching for solutions to these questions for years and now appear to have found some answers. Probably the best place to start considering the problem is with the teeth themselves and their structure.

Every tooth has a crown of dentin covered with enamel, the hardest substance in the body. It also has a neck and a root. The neck of the tooth is the area between the crown and the root. The outer surface of the root is cementum which is not as hard as enamel but rather is similar to dentin. At the center of the root is the pulp cavity containing nerves, lymph and blood vessels, and some enzymes.

The life of a tooth is divided into three periods: (1) development—crown forming and calcifying in the jaw; (2) maturation—erupting into the mouth, and forming roots; and (3) maintenance.

Like the bones, teeth are composed largely of minerals—chiefly calcium, phosphorus, magnesium, and carbon. Other elements, too, are present in minute amounts, such as fluorine, tin, zinc, iron, strontium, titanium, vanadium, chromium, platinum, and silver. Add to these protein, lipids, water, and oxygen. Vitamins A, C, and D, while not part of the teeth, are needed for their proper development.

Anything that favors tooth decay is said to be cariogenic; that which hinders it, cariostatic.

Dental disease may involve any part of the tooth or gums. When diseased or damaged, the teeth cannot repair themselves as the bones are able to. Thus preventing dental disease is more desirable and much less painful than curing it. The early deciduous or "milk" teeth should be given the best possible care, since this helps to ensure better formed and healthier permanent teeth.

Few people are born with "perfect" teeth and fewer maintain a healthy set throughout life. Many factors are involved in the development of sound teeth and in their preservation. Among them are inheritance, nutrition and food habits, oral environment, and fluorine.

Inheritance

Your grandparents and your great-grandparents have influenced the health and formation of your mouth. You inherit from them resistance or susceptibility of your teeth to decay, as well as their size and form. In animal experiments it has been possible to develop caries-susceptible and caries-resistant strains of white rats. Heredity appears to give human beings teeth either resistant or susceptible to cavities.

The experiences of Eskimo tribes and some other primitive peoples have shown that what appears to be heredity may be modified. As long as they continued on their traditional diets they were caries-free, but as soon as they adopted the refined foods of civilization, dental disease followed.

Your mother's diet before you were born also had its part in determining the soundness of your teeth. The deciduous teeth are formed in the jaw before birth. If your mother had adequate nutrition in all respects, your chance of avoiding dental troubles is greater.

Nutrition and Food Habits

Repeated experimental studies have demonstrated the effect of adequate nutrition, with emphasis on specific nutrients and food habits on the incidence of caries.

A diet which is patterned after the Daily Food Guide helps to ensure adequate nutrition. This should provide ample protein, minerals, and vitamins.

The teeth are made up largely of calcium and phosphorus; so it is to be expected that they will suffer if the diet is low in either. The calcium:phosphorus ratio, along with vitamin D, particularly affects the enamel and the dentin.

Lady May Mellanby more than fifty years ago reported studies on vitamin D and teeth in *The Lancet,* a British medical journal. She used puppies as experimental animals. If the mother dog's diet was deficient in vitamin D, the structure of the puppies' deciduous teeth was defective and eruption time was delayed. If the puppies themselves lacked vitamin D, it affected their permanent teeth—the enamel and dentin, the time they "cut" their teeth, and their position in the jaw.

Lady Mellanby also examined the teeth of school children in England at intervals for a number of years and discovered a high correlation between vitamin D and the structure of the teeth and number of cavities. She noted that sunshine and cod liver oil, both good sources of vitamin D, were closely related to the health of the teeth.

Research indicates that fewer cavities result when diets conducive to the development of tooth decay are supplemented with phosphate.

In one study five hundred school children, five to sixteen years of age, were divided into two groups. The first group was given presweetened cereal with added phosphate; the second group received presweetened cereal without phosphate. The first group had 20 to 40 percent fewer cavities.

In 1967 the effect of adding phosphate to chewing gum was reported. One group of children received chewing gum sweetened with sugar; another, gum with sugar and phosphate; and a third group, sugarless gum. At the end of two and one half years, the children chewing the sugar gum had more caries than the other two groups. The number of cavities of those chewing sugarless or sugar-phosphate gum was about the same. This would seem to indicate that the effect of the phosphate was to reduce cavities.

It is believed that phosphates may be the protective substances lacking in refined diets. A number of studies suggest that loss of phosphates during milling of cereals and the refinement of sugar may be the causative factor in dental caries. A person who includes moderate amounts of milk and unrefined cereals and bread in his diet and avoids too many sweets such as "soda pop" and candies will probably consume an adequate amount of phosphates. Other foods high in phosphates are dried beans, peas, and other legumes and nuts, especially peanuts and Brazil nuts.

In animal studies, rats on low protein diets were found to be more susceptible to caries. In other research, supplementing rats' diets with the amino acid lysine prevented decay. While results of animal experiments do not always apply to humans, it is known that sufficient protein is essential to good nutrition, which in turn will benefit the teeth.

Vitamins A, C, and D are especially associated with tooth formation. Vitamin C deficiency is believed to be one of the causes of periodontal disease which affects the gums and bony structures of the teeth. Vitamin B_6 appears to be important in the post-eruptive period of the tooth.

Sugar and candy have long been indicted as cavity producers. According to the American Dental Association, carbonated soft drinks, sweet sticky foods, candy-coated chewing gum, and breath mints are all major causes of dental decay. Other refined carbohydrates may also produce cavities.

Dr. James H. Shaw writing in *Nutrition in Health and Disease* (1968) by Wohl and Goodhard states, "There can be no question that the excessive consumption of carbohydrate-containing foods, especially those that are retained on the tooth surfaces, is responsible to a large degree for a high dental caries incidence in caries-susceptible populations. . . . As the availability and frequency of carbohydrate consumption increases, the potentiality for the development and progression of caries increases."—Page 647.

Many studies have been reported on the effect of refined carbohydrates, and sugar in particular, on the teeth. An interesting one comes from Switzerland. The number of decayed, missing, or filled teeth per individual was compared with the diet of over ten thousand inhabitants of mountain farms in nine regions of Switzerland. As an example of the findings, the incidence of decaying teeth was greater among school children in one region where there was higher intake of sugar and refined carbohydrates, than that of children in another region who ate less refined carbohydrate and sugar.

The frequency of eating has a bearing on caries formation. It can almost be said, the fewer the meals the fewer the cavities. Eating between meals and frequent snacking is detrimental to the teeth. Even candy and other sweets have been found to be less harmful, if eaten in larger amounts less often and if eaten with meals rather than between meals.

It is small wonder that teen-agers tend to have caries, since they are inveterate snackers and heavy refined carbohydrate eaters. A market study has revealed that teen-agers, who make up about one seventh of the population, eat one-third of all the candy bars consumed in the United States. And what about the many soft drinks and malts?

Exclusive use of soft foods is not desirable. The teeth to be healthy need something to chew on. What dentists call detergent foods are recommended. They are crisp raw vegetables and fruits and moderately hard foods, such as dried toast, which require chewing. These have been called nature's toothbrushes.

The Oral Environment

Bacteria are agents in tooth decay. If the mouth could be kept free of microorganisms, there would be no cavities. This is hardly possible with humans, but it has been done with animals. Caries-susceptible rats were kept germ-free, and they did not develop cavities even when they were fed a ration high in sugar.

Bacteria must have carbohydrate to produce caries. The amount of sugar or carbohydrate is less important, however, than the time they are in the mouth and the frequency of eating them.

A California Dental Association leaflet entitled "Your Teeth" states: "Research has shown that sugar undoubtedly plays a major role in dental decay. Bacteria normally present in the mouth, feed on sugar products and within minutes produce an acid which attacks tooth enamel. This process, repeated over and over, leads to tooth decay."

The saliva has a protective effect. It has been found that when the salivary glands are removed there is a marked increase of caries. It is important to chew the food thoroughly, as that stimulates the flow of saliva.

Fluoridation

In some areas of Texas and Colorado the people were troubled with mottled teeth and it was found to be caused by the high fluoride content of the water. Interestingly, they had no dental caries. This led to further investigation and finally the suggestion of adding minute amounts of fluoride to food or water.

Fluoridation of water suggested itself as the simplest method of reducing cavities. There has been considerable controversy over this since fluoride is a substance that is poisonous when used in too large amounts. The same is true of some other trace minerals and a few of the vitamins, however; and no one fears using them.

One to one and one half parts per million (ppm) of fluoride has been used in fluoridation of water. This ratio controls cavities and is far below the toxic level. In some areas there is naturally 8 to 12 ppm in water, and there are no harmful effects except the unattractive mottling of the teeth.

About sixty million people in three thousand communities are drinking fluoridated water and nearly eight million additional people live where the water is naturally high in fluorides.

Dr. Donald Fraser in discussing nutrition problems in North America at the Western Hemisphere Nutrition Congress in 1965 stated that caries incidence could be cut in half with fluoridation of water.

Dr. J. M. Dunning reported in the *New England Medical Journal* that caries were reduced 50 to 70 percent among youth whose teeth were formed after fluoridation.

Fluoride in toothpaste probably has some beneficial effects. But it is quickly diluted with water and washed away. Thus it remains in the mouth such a short time that its benefits are believed to be minimal. It has been found that fluoride is also lost from toothpaste to some extent during storage.

Fluoride in water and in food has been found to reduce cavities and has not proved harmful to date if used in the minute quantities suggested.

In Summary

For fewer (or no) cavities:

1. Follow the Daily Food Guide.
2. Make every meal nutritious with ample protein, high vitamins and minerals, especially vitamins A, C, and D, and calcium and phosphorus.
3. Do not eat between meals; especially avoid snacking on high carbohydrate foods.
4. Eat every day some of the detergent foods—nature's toothbrushes.
5. If candy is to be eaten, eat it only at meals and never between meals.
6. Because of their natural phosphate content, unrefined breads and cereals should be chosen.
7. Drink fluoridated water.
8. Keep the teeth clean.
9. Have periodic checks with your dentist.

Parents-to-Be

Brenda and Bob were expecting their first baby and felt thrilled and awed at the prospect. What a privilege it would be to raise this child, and how great was their responsibility to ensure it a good mind and healthy body!

"How can we give our baby a good start in life? What can we do to safeguard his health?" they asked their obstetrician. If you are a parent-to-be, you will find the information the doctor gave them helpful to you too.

He told them that though pregnancy is a normal process, there are many complex metabolic and physiologic changes that take place within the body.

"The factors involved are often complicated and difficult to interpret, and it is apparent that nutrition plays a vital role," he said.

"Dr. Genevieve Stearns has worked with mothers and children for many years at the University of Iowa Medical Center," he told them, "and she has said that 'the best insurance for a healthy infant is a mother who is healthy and well-nourished throughout her entire life as well as during pregnancy itself.'

"Diet during pregnancy usually reflects lifetime food habits," he continued. "If yours have been good, you can be thankful. If they have been poor, you cannot change the past; but you can begin today to improve your nutritional state and general health by choosing an adequate diet and observing good health practices. After the diet is improved, it takes time for the body to realize the real benefits, however, even with the increased ability during pregnancy to utilize nutrients. A study reports that girls who had subsisted on poor diets, required five months, after changing to adequate diets, to utilize and retain the same amount of calcium as did consistently well-fed girls.

"Studies have shown that improving the diet during pregnancy influences the health and vigor of the new-born infant and affects the way the mother comes through delivery and the length of her recovery period. If the nutritional state of the mother remains good, the health of the infants in successive pregnancies is better."

Dr. Calvin showed them a graphic picture (Figure 1) of the effect of diet during pregnancy on new-born infants.

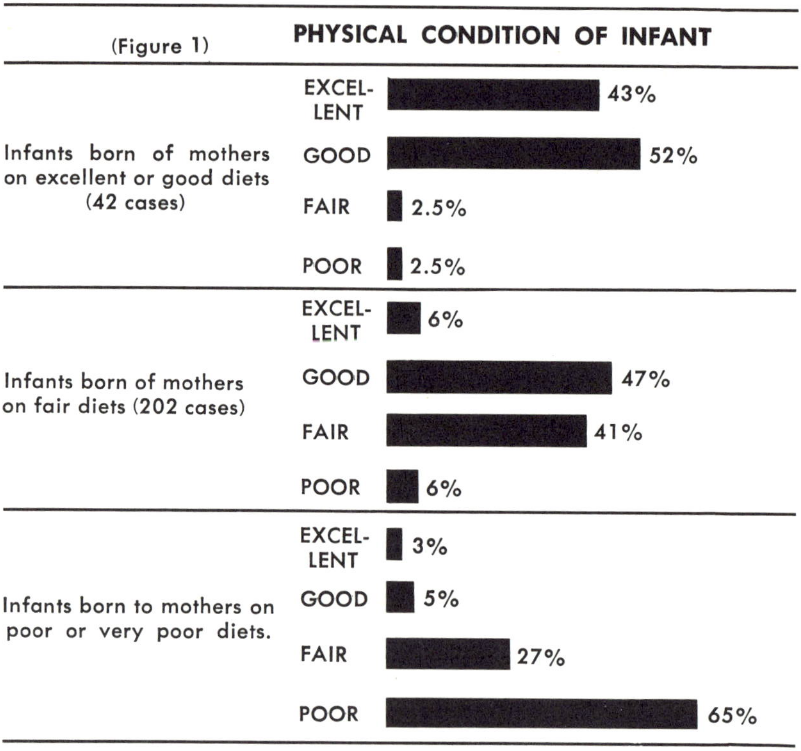

The relation of the prenatal diet of the mothers to the condition of the infant at birth. Note the increase in poor ratings of the infants as the diets go from good to very poor.

(Adapted from Burke, B.S. et al.: *American Journal of Nutrition,* 38:453, 1949.)

Much was learned about nutrition and pregnancy during World War II, he told them. It was noticed that malnutrition increased the risk of unhealthy offspring; that good nutrition before and during pregnancy resulted in healthier, stronger babies and less risk of premature births, stillbirths, or malformations.

During the long siege of Leningrad, when the food supply was both insufficient and of poor quality, the birth rate fell markedly, prematurity increased 41 percent, and a third of the premature infants died during their first month. Even the full-term babies that survived nursed poorly and had low vitality and lowered resistance to infections.

In the British Isles where, during the entire war years, special attention was given to the diets of pregnant women, there was a significant drop in the infant death rate and an increase in the health ratings of the new-born.

Bob had read that a baby is born every eight seconds in the United States. He estimated that was 11,000 new Americans a day and that it could add to the population each month a city the size of Syracuse, New York, or every year one the size of Chicago. Yet, the article said, the infant mortality rate is higher in the United States than in fourteen other countries. That disturbed him, since America is regarded as one of the most favored nations in the world. When he asked the doctor about it, his answer was, "Affluence and an abundance of available food do not always mean good nutrition or wise health practices."

Brenda and Bob were told that the first eight to twelve weeks of pregnancy is a period in the development of the baby-to-be when it is most susceptible to unfavorable conditions and a time when the possibility of abortion is greatest. In this period nausea and vomiting, sometimes called morning sickness, is quite common and if severe and persistent, should be treated by a physician.

"During the first trimester of pregnancy it is not necessary to increase your food intake. If your diet before pregnancy measured up to the recommendations of the National Research Council, you should be receiving a good supply of the essential nutrients," Brenda was told. In subsequent visits to the doctor she learned much more and was given a daily food guide, basic meal pattern, and menus. (Note pages 140-143.) You, too, will find these helpful as you plan for your baby-to-be.

During the second and third trimesters of pregnancy, the National Research Council recommends an increase in almost all the essential nutrients as well as calories. If you nurse your baby, an even greater increase is indicated. These recommended allowances are listed below and are contrasted with the requirements of an average woman eighteen to thirty-five years of age.

RECOMMENDED DIETARY ALLOWANCES (Revised 1968)

	Non-Pregnancy	Pregnancy	Lactation
Calories	2000	2200	3000
Protein, grams	55	65	75
Vitamin A value, I.U.	5000	6000	8000
Vitamin D, I.U.	400 (18-22 yrs.)	400	400
Vitamin E, I.U.	25	30	30
Ascorbic Acid, Mg.	55	60	60
Folacin, Mg.	0.4	0.8	0.5
Niacin Equiv., Mg.	13	15	20
Riboflavin, Mg.	1.5	1.8	2.0
Thiamine, Mg.	1.0	1.1	1.5
Vitamin B_6, Mg.	2.0	2.5	2.5
Vitamin B_{12}, Mcg.	5	8	6
Calcium, grams	0.8	1.2	1.3
Phosphorus, grams	0.8	1.2	1.3
Iodine, Mcg.	100	125	150
Iron, Mg.	18	18	18
Magnesium, Mg.	300-350	450	450

These recommended increases should be met if the suggested additions in the Daily Food Guide (pages 140-143) are included in the diet. The menu pattern and sample menus show the simple adjustments necessary to add more calories. It is also obvious that more than adequate protein may be easily included on a lacto-ovo-vegetarian diet.

The 200-calorie increase recommended during pregnancy is sufficient to care for your increase in metabolism without causing excessive weight gain. The extra calories and protein are easily supplied by the additions of milk and the increased amounts of vegetables and fruits indicated.

A program of reducing should not be undertaken except under the direction of your attending physician and never at your own discretion, as complications may result. If it is necessary for any reason to lose weight during pregnancy, the calories may be decreased providing there are sufficient protein, minerals, and vitamins in the diet. But it is doubtful that enough minerals and vitamins can be furnished when your diet is decreased below 1500 calories, without supplementation.

A gain of not more than eighteen to twenty-two pounds during your entire pregnancy is normal. Ideally your gain in weight will be gradual and regular in about the following way: one and a half pounds the first ten weeks with a total of about three pounds by the end of the fourth month, and then a gain of about 0.8 pounds a week the remainder of the time. Insufficient gain in weight is as undesirable as excessive weight gain. Both are associated with increased possibility of a premature birth or toxemia.

A liberal intake of protein and minerals is essential for the formation of the teeth and bony structure of your baby, for the growth and development of your mammary tissues, and for a reserve for the stresses of delivery and milk production. The protein content of the diet is usually considered a good index to the other nutrients. If your diet is low in protein, the other essentials are often in short supply. It has been observed that the hemoglobin of a mother-to-be is higher and there is less edema when protein is liberally provided.

An increase in calcium safeguards your health and bony structures during pregnancy and furnishes an ample supply for the bony framework and teeth of your developing baby. Then, too, if you receive ample calcium, you will be more capable of nursing. Three or four cups of milk a day during pregnancy and one quart or more during lactation will supply most of the calcium needed.

Ample iron in the diet is a safeguard against anemia because of blood loss during delivery. In the period of pregnancy, the baby also builds up a reserve supply of iron for use during the first months of life when milk, which is low in iron, is his chief source of nourishment. To ensure sufficient iron intake, an egg should be included in the diet daily, with a liberal use of green leafy vegetables, whole grains, legumes, some nuts, and some dried fruits as prunes, figs, dates, and apricots.

Pronounced deficiencies of iodine during pregnancy may cause goiter and in some instances cretinism (failure of the infant to develop mentally and to grow normally). The use of iodized salt is suggested for those living in areas where the water supply and soil are deficient in iodine.

If your diet is increased to meet the protein and mineral needs, the vitamin requirements, with the exception of vitamin D, should be met. In some instances the vitamin needs of an infant will take priority over the needs of its mother.

There is no substitute for a good diet habitually followed, but it is not the only factor in ensuring the health of the baby. Mental attitude, emotions, and living habits may affect the baby for good or ill. Discontent, worry, grief, fear, excitement, overfatigue, insufficient sleep, irregularity, intemperance—all have an adverse effect.

The influence of emotional upsets was shown in one study by a prompt decrease in calcium retention. The decrease tended to parallel the degree of the emotional disturbance, and this occurred regardless of the character of the previous diet. Other studies have shown similar effects in connection with other nutrients.

"The relation that exists between the mind and the body is very intimate. . . . The condition of the mind affects the health to a far greater degree than many realize. . . .

"Courage, hope, faith, sympathy, love promote health and prolong life. A contented mind, a cheerful spirit, is health to the body and strength to the soul." These statements from the book *The Ministry of Healing,* by E. G. White, page 241, apply with special force during pregnancy and lactation.

After the Baby Arrives

Mother's milk is the baby's best food. It is just the right temperature, easily digested, economical, and usually free from harmful bacteria.

For the first three or four days it contains a substance called colostrum which is of special value to the new baby as it has more protein, acts as a laxative, and contains antibodies which help resist infection. Some of these qualities stay in the milk for as long as two weeks.

Nursing your baby is important for another reason. As you cuddle and nurse him, you give him a sense of security and belonging by the intimacy of the relationship you establish with him. If nursing your baby is not possible, however, do not be unduly concerned. You can still love and cuddle him. Many bottle-fed babies have grown up feeling secure and wanted. While artificial feeding is not as desirable as breast feeding, there are excellent formulas. Successful methods for artificial feeding have been available for years.

The baby grows faster during his first year of life than he will ever grow again. This makes extra demands on you as long as you are nursing him, since you must eat enough to maintain your own health and to nourish a rapidly growing infant.

The reason some women have more milk than others is not clearly understood; but it is known that a calm, well-nourished mother has a much better chance of feeding her child. To increase milk production include daily four or more glasses of milk in your own diet. Drink plenty of fluids (one to two quarts of water and fruit juice daily). And use a liberal supply of foods rich in vitamins, which are believed to stimulate milk production.

Eat plenty of wholesome food prepared in a plain and simple way. Avoid such things as fried foods, pickles, and highly spiced or seasoned foods. If you are having difficulty eating sufficient food, try wheat germ and brewer's yeast. They may increase your appetite and are excellent sources of the B-complex vitamins.

Worry, excitement, over-fatigue, digestive disturbances, and constipation tend to diminish the milk flow and may also have a disturbing influence upon the infant.

To nurse your baby successfully demands a calm, happy spirit, a quiet, contented life, moderate exercise in the fresh air, pleasant work, periods of rest and relaxation both physical and mental, and an intelligent choice of the most nourishing food.

DAILY FOOD GUIDE

	Non-Pregnant	Pregnant	Lactating
Protein Food	2 or more servings, including legumes, cheese, nuts, vegetable proteins, eggs, 3-4 times weekly	2 or more servings, including 1 egg, daily	3 or more servings, including 1 egg, daily
Milk	2 cups or more	3 cups or more	4 cups or more
Vegetables and Fruits	4 servings or more, cooked or raw, including: Dark green, leafy, and deep yellow vegetables Potatoes and other vegetables	5 servings, cooked or raw	6 servings, cooked or raw
	Citrus fruit or juice or tomatoes	Same	Same and 3 cups fruit juice 4-6 cups water
Bread and Cereal	4 or more servings Whole grain, enriched or restored ½ cup cooked cereal = 1 slice bread	Same	Same (May increase if weight gain needed)
Fat	To meet body's need	Same	Same
Extras	Fruit or simple dessert to meet calorie needs	Same	Same

USE FOOD THAT ADDS EXTRA MINERALS AND VITAMINS, AVOID THOSE THAT SUPPLY CALORIES ONLY.

BASIC MEAL PATTERN*

Non-Pregnant	Pregnant	Lactating
BREAKFAST	**BREAKFAST**	**BREAKFAST**
Citrus fruit or juice	Citrus Juice	Citrus juice
Fruit	Fruit	Fruit
Cereal	Cereal	Cereal
Toast	Egg	Egg
Milk and/or egg	Toast	Toast
	Milk	Milk—2 cups
DINNER	**DINNER**	**DINNER**
Protein dish	Protein dish	Protein dish
Dark green leafy or deep yellow vegetable	Dark green leafy or deep yellow vegetable—2 servings†	Dark green leafy or yellow vegetable—2 servings
Potato or other vegetable	Potato or other vegetable	Potato or other vegetable
Salad	Salad	Salad—2 servings
Bread	Bread	Bread
	Milk	Milk
LUNCH OR SUPPER	**LUNCH OR SUPPER**	**LUNCH OR SUPPER**
Protein dish or cream soup	Protein dish or cream soup	Protein dish or cream soup
Fruit and/or vegetable	Fruit and/or vegetable	Vegetable
Bread	Bread	Bread
Milk	Milk	Milk

*The basic meal pattern does not include fats and extras. Such foods may be added to round out the diet to meet the caloric needs but should not replace the foods listed.

†A serving of vegetable or fruit is considered at ½ cup cooked or ⅔ cup raw.

SAMPLE MENUS

Non-Pregnant	Pregnant		Lactation
1800 Calories 78 gm. Protein	2000 Calories 78 gm. Protein	2200 Calories 84 gm. Protein	3000 Calories 104 gm. Protein
BREAKFAST	**BREAKFAST**	**BREAKFAST**	**BREAKFAST**
Orange juice—1 cup	Orange juice—1 cup	Orange juice—1 cup	Orange juice—1 cup
Stewed prunes—6 medium and 3 tbsp. juice	Stewed prunes—6 medium and 3 tbsp. juice	Stewed prunes—6 medium and 3 tbsp. juice	Stewed prunes—6 medium and 3 tbsp. juice
Roman Meal—2⁄3 cup and 1 tbsp. wheat germ	Roman meal—2⁄3 cup and 1 tbsp. wheat germ	Roman Meal—2⁄3 cup and 1 tbsp. wheat germ	Roman Meal—2⁄3 cup and 1 tbsp. wheat germ
Poached egg (large) Whole wheat toast	Poached egg (large) Whole wheat toast	Poached egg (large) Whole wheat toast	Poached egg (large) Whole wheat toast
		Margarine—1 tsp.	Margarine—1 tsp.
		Honey—1 tbsp.	Honey—1 tbsp.
Milk—1 cup	Milk—1 cup	Milk—1 cup	Milk—1 1⁄2 cup
DINNER	**DINNER**	**DINNER**	**DINNER**
†Princess loaf with mushroom Gravy Quik	†Princess loaf with mushroom Gravy Quik	†Princess loaf with mushroom Gravy Quik	†Princess loaf with mushroom Gravy Quik
Baked potato—large	Baked potato—large	Baked potato—large	Baked potato—large
Spinach and mustard greens—1 cup cooked, lemon	Spinach and mustard greens—1 cup cooked, lemon	Spinach and mustard greens—1 cup cooked, lemon	Spinach and mustard greens—1 1⁄2 cup cooked, lemon
Margarine—1 tbsp.	Margarine—1 tbsp.	Margarine—1 tbsp.	Margarine—1 tbsp.
Lettuce and tomato salad —1 cup	Lettuce and tomato salad —1 cup	Lettuce and tomato salad —1 cup	Lettuce and tomato salad —1 cup
	Thousand Island dressing —1 tbsp.	Thousand Island dressing —1 tbsp.	Thousand Island dressing —1 tbsp.
		Oatmeal cookies—2	Oatmeal cookies—2
Skim or buttermilk—1 cup	Skim or buttermilk—1 cup	Skim or buttermilk—1 cup	Milk or buttermilk— 1 1⁄2 cup

(SAMPLE MENUS—Continued)

SUPPER	SUPPER	SUPPER	SUPPER
†Cottage cheese souffle	†Cottage cheese souffle	†Cottage cheese souffle	†Cottage cheese souffle
Whole grain bread—1 slice	Whole grain bread—1 slice	Whole grain bread—1 slice	Whole grain bread—2 slices
Margarine—1 tsp.	Margarine—1 tsp.	Margarine—1 tsp.	Margarine—1½ tsp.
Fresh, sliced peaches or apricots—1 cup	Fresh, sliced peaches or apricots—1 cup	Fresh, sliced peaches or apricots—1 cup	Fresh, sliced peaches or apricots—1 cup
Milk—1 cup	Dried figs—3 large	Dried figs—3 large	Dried figs—3 large
	Milk—1 cup	Milk—1 cup	Milk—1 cup
			Between meals—3 cups of pineapple, grape, tomato, or orange juice

†Recipes for these dishes can be found in the companion cookbook series to this volume, *Vegetarian Cookery*.

"As the Twig Is Bent"

Marcus Aurelius Afortunatus Tidd was a storybook character. And no matter how many years have passed since we last read the story, he always remains vivid in our minds. Marcus was a fat boy, and he had one sport and one accomplishment—eating. The other children watched with envy and amazement as he gorged on bananas by the dozen, uncounted cookies, and any amount of cake or pie or ice cream—anytime! Most amazing, there was an unlimited supply and no one to say No!

His fate was not part of the story, but unless he quickly and drastically changed his food habits, it does not take a crystal ball to predict it. As a result of his eating habits Marcus Aurelius was suffering from a common form of malnutrition, overweight. He had no nutritional bulwark against the disease and infection that would plague him regularly. He was destined to make frequent and painful visits to the dentist and early lose his teeth. Poor Marcus Aurelius Afortunatus Tidd; because of his undesirable nutritional practices, his chances for a long, healthy, and happy life were nil.

Ensuring sound nutritional practices during the period of growth is of particular consequence since these are the foundation years. These are the years when "the twig is bent." A child may be malnourished and, like Marcus Aurelius, have an abundance of food. It is not just the quantity but the kind of food your child eats that counts. How important it is, then, to study not only how much to feed him, but what and how to feed him! Become familiar with the criteria of a healthy child: normal weight; well-developed muscles; strong, straight bones; sound teeth; good posture; clear, ruddy complexion; shiny hair; sparkling eyes; alert mind; vitality and energy; and freedom from disease.

Just as a young tree bent crooked cannot straighten when it is older, so effort and care later in life cannot entirely overcome the effects of poor nutritional practices in childhood. Dr. Philip L. White in an address to the American School Health Association put it this way:

"It has been established in studies in most every country of the world that interference with growth and development during the first four years will produce very significant stunting of growth and in all probability also stunting of mental development. . . . It is now evident that if the nutritional setback occurs before the fourth year, even though the child recovers and is essentially a normal individual, he never makes up that difference."

Unfortunately, many children, even in the United States with its abundance, are getting poor materials with which to build for the future.

Although an infant or child may not develop marked symptoms, he still can be suffering from the effects of malnutrition. Iron deficiency anemia, for instance, is prevalent in infants and preschool children in some areas. Illnesses, particularly upper respiratory tract infections, are one of the results. In the *American Journal of Clinical Nutrition,* Dr. Elinor F. Downs states that "even a slight deficiency of protein intake during the first three years of life when growth demands are high may lead to precarious nutritional imbalance, and if prolonged it can cause irreversible changes in both physical growth and mental development."

We have seen that children need the same nutrients as adults, and the Daily Food Guide can be followed in planning the meals for the whole family. Your child's protein, mineral, vitamin, and energy requirements per unit of weight, however, are higher than an adult's. A normal healthy child needs considerably more energy food for his size because he is much more active than an adult and his basal metabolic rate (energy used to keep body processes operating) is higher. This does not mean that he should be given large quantities of food or unlimited amounts of "empty calories" such as refined sugars in the form of candy and desserts. He needs the minerals and vitamins which are in good wholesome food and absent in "empty calorie" foods.

In planning your family's diet, thought should be given to the differences in digestive ability of small children. A little child needs simple, easily digested food. Such items as rich pastries and sweets, sauces, gravies, fried foods, pickles, and highly seasoned foods are best omitted from the whole family's bill of fare and particularly from your child's. It scarcely needs to be said that coffee, tea, cola drinks, and alcoholic beverages should never be given to children.

The foundation years may be divided into three categories: infancy, the first two years; preschool, two to five; and the elementary school age, six to twelve years.

During the first year your baby's food schedule is usually under the direction of a physician. He suggests when and what foods to add to his diet. By the end of the first year, he is usually getting cereal and toast, pureed vegetables, stewed fruits, ripe bananas, orange juice, egg and other simple protein foods, and of course milk. During the second year additional foods are introduced and vegetables are served chopped, and in time, whole. The diet is kept simple but increased in quantity and variety.

The preschool years are often the most neglected nutritionally, although their importance cannot be overemphasized. During these years continue to increase quantities of food and give more solid food. The diet should consist of milk, eggs, fruits, vegetables, cereals and bread, and simple protein foods. Children of this age are usually fond of crisp raw vegetables, such as carrot sticks, celery hearts, and cabbage and lettuce wedges, which they can hold in their fingers.

When the child starts to school, his nutritional practices will affect not only his general health, but his success in school. Fortunately for children who do not otherwise get an adequate diet, the school lunch program with its Grade A lunch insures at least one good meal five days a week.

First in the list of food to supply your child's needs is milk. He should have the equivalent of two to four cups of milk a day, depending upon his age. If he dislikes milk, it may be used in soups, drinks, simple desserts, cereals, and other dishes—the important point being that he get the milk. For safety's sake it should be pasteurized or sterilized. It may be fresh, dried, canned, or in the form of milk products such as cheese and ice cream. Soybean milk may be used, but unless fortified it is deficient in calcium and does not contain vitamin B_{12}.

Occasionally a child will develop such a fondness for milk that he will prefer it to other foods. Parents have in some instances encouraged this to the child's detriment. Milk is important in his diet for it is an excellent source of calcium and contains good protein and other nutrients; but it is low in iron, bulk, and some other needed factors. A child needs a variety of foods.

Two or more servings of protein-rich food such as cheese, eggs, dried legumes (peas and beans), nuts and nut butters should be a part of his daily diet. Soybeans and garbanzos are nearly equivalent to meat in protein value, but the protein of most other legumes rates lower than meat. Their protein value may be improved by combination with cereals and breads. Three or four eggs a week should usually be included.

Most children are fond of peanut butter. In fact, it is customary to speak of the peanut butter age. Peanut butter is a good source of protein and niacin. Two level tablespoons of peanut butter supply about the same amount of protein as one ounce of cooked, lean meat. Peanut butter should be used in moderation, however, since it is a concentrated food high in fat.

Children like fruit, and at least two servings should be included in the diet daily. A glass of juice such as orange or tomato may be part of breakfast or a nourishment at midmorning or midafternoon. Three or more servings of vegetables, including green leafy or yellow ones, at least three times a week should be part of the day's menu. Vegetables may be made attractive to children in various ways. Greens may be served in fancy molds, made firm with agar or gelatin. Raw vegetables such as carrot curls, celery sticks, radish roses, cauliflowerettes, mild turnip slices, and cherry tomatoes often are more acceptable than the cooked. These and fresh fruits are rich sources of vitamin C as well as other nutrients.

Bread and cereals should be either whole grain or enriched. A certain amount of fat is needed in the diet, but because it is customarily supplied in more than adequate amounts, it is not mentioned in most daily food guides.

During the first few years a child is constantly being introduced to new foods. The way they are presented and the attitudes of other members of the family will have much to do with their acceptance. Introduce them gradually in small quantities. If he dislikes the food, do not make an issue of it. Withdraw it and plan to include it later in a different form. Remember he is small; so do not expect him to eat large amounts. Give him small servings and an opportunity for seconds if he wishes.

Mealtime should be a happy time. Try to avoid disciplining your child during the meal. He should not eat when emotionally upset or when over-tired or excited. Do not make the small child and his eating or refusing to eat the center of attention. He will quickly learn that he can get attention this way or by dawdling over his food. Quietly remove the food and let him wait until the next meal for more. He will not starve or be permanently injured if he misses a few meals. Ordinarily unless he is ill, and if no fuss is made and he does not sense your concern, he will soon begin eating as he should. If he continues to eat poorly, consult your pediatrician.

Good breakfasts are essential to your child's health and success. Children who come to school without breakfast are not as alert and tire more quickly. A good day starts with a good breakfast.

Snacks have come to be a part of the American way of life. While the child should not be constantly munching on tidbits, regular snack times may be a beneficial part of the program for some children. Nourishing foods supplying minerals, vitamins, and other nutrients may substitute for "empty calorie" snacks, but avoid heavy foods that take the child's appetite for meals. Such foods as fruit juice, fresh fruit, or graham crackers and milk make light and appetizing but nourishing snacks. It should be emphasized that snack times should be at regular hours just as mealtimes are.

A suggested day's program outlined for the different ages of childhood follows. Some children will eat considerably more than others, and the plan allows for flexibility.

In summary, infancy and childhood are the foundation years—the years when the twig is bent. The future health of your child, even the length of his life, may be affected by his nutrition during these years. When planning his diet ensure first the important nutrients found in milk, protein-rich foods, vegetables, fruits, fruit juices, and whole grain or enriched cereals and bread. These are essential for a strong foundation of health. After the food essentials are supplied, the extras may be added. They, too, can be planned to add to the nutritional value of the diet and thus help in building a good foundation for a long and healthy life. "As the twig is bent" during these foundation years, the future health will be determined.

SUGGESTED DAILY PROGRAM FOR CHILDREN 1-12 YEARS

Food	**Infancy 1-2 years**	**Preschool 2-5 years**	**Elementary School 6-12 years**
Milk	2-3 cups	2-3 cups	2-4 cups
Protein-rich food	2 (1-oz. each)	2 (2-oz. each)	2 (4-oz. each)
Egg	½	1 daily or 4 times/week	I daily or 4 times/week
Potatoes or equivalent	½—1 small or 2 tbsp.	1 small or 3-4 tbsp.	1 medium or 4-6 tbsp.
Green leafy or deep yellow vegetables	2-3 tbsp.	3-4 tbsp. cooked or 2-3 small raw pieces	½-⅔ cup
Other vegetable	2-3 tbsp.	As above	Increased quantity
Citrus, tomato, melon, or other vitamin C food	½ cup	½ cup or 1 med. orange	1 cup or 1 large orange
Other fruit	2-4 tbsp.	¼-½ cup	½-1 cup
Cereal, whole grain, etc.	4-6 tbsp.	½ cup or more	¾-1 cup
Bread, whole grain or enriched	1-2 slices	2-3 slices	2-4 slices or more
Margarine or other fat	1 tbsp.	1 tbsp.	1 tbsp. or more
Dessert	Preferably fruit or simple desserts 2-3 tbsp.	¼-½ cup	½-1 cup

Teen Fare

In a certain country, six out of every ten teen-age girls and four out of every ten boys are reported to be physically below par because of impoverished diets. Is that country India? Africa? China? No, it's the United States, the most affluent country in the world. The diets of most teen-agers in this country are short of calcium, iron, and vitamin C.

Why do so many teen-agers have poor dietary habits? Are you concerned about the teen-agers in your family? A look at the physical demands during the teen years and some typical teen-age habits may help to answer the question.

The years from twelve to nineteen are the link between childhood and adulthood. They are a time of intense physical and emotional change. The adolescent, while rapidly maturing physically, is also developing individuality, self-expression, and independence. He rejects anything that savors of "kid stuff." What his teen peers do and say is more impressive than any adult admonitions. There is a strong "togetherness" with other teen-agers who dress alike, comb their hair alike, talk alike, listen to the same records, and enjoy the same kinds of food eaten at the same times and places.

Teen-agers tend to be snackers. It is a habit and, unless the snack is wisely chosen, a problem. To them "snack time" is a social time when they get together with other teen-agers. They frequently eat one to three snacks daily, and it is estimated that they consume about a third or a fourth of their total calories in this way. Snacks can be wholesome and can make a nutritious and sizable contribution to the day's diet. Too often, however, they are mostly "empty calories," satisfying the appetite so there is no hunger for more nutritious foods.

The fewer calories in a day's diet, the more essential it is that any snacks eaten supply good amounts of nutrients. Because teen-age girls require fewer calories, choosing "empty calories" at snack time is more serious for them than for boys who can easily eat almost 1,000 calories more in a day.

Snacking is not a desirable habit for most teen-agers, although some may benefit from more than the three meals. They may need the additional calories. If nutritious, appetizing meals including some of the teen-ager's favorite foods are served at regular times, there will be less tendency to snack. There is another side to teen-age snacking. Snacking during the teen years may establish habits that carry over into the adult years when such habits cause obesity and other problems.

A survey of snacking choices of 6,200 students in North Carolina revealed that those in grades 10 to 12 usually chose soft drinks, candy, or other sweets, while the seventh to ninth graders picked more nourishing foods such as milk, fruit, bread, and cereal. The evening snack of the older youth consisted of more of the same type of refreshment as that eaten earlier in the day, although milk was included now and then. This pointed up the fact that in North Carolina at least, the older the teen-ager, the poorer the snacking habits.

Missing meals is another teen-age problem. Breakfast is most frequently skipped, but a sizable minority of teen-agers miss not only breakfast but one other meal. In the Los Angeles area, it was discovered, some teen-agers never have even one well-organized meal a day. A survey of a teen-age group in Idaho revealed that 6 percent of them missed breakfasts, 6 percent missed dinners, and 12 percent missed lunches.

Breakfast is a most important meal that should contribute one-fourth to one-third of the day's requirements. Breakfast eaters are more alert, more resistant to fatigue, more efficient. This efficiency, so the studies show, applies to scholastic performance as well as work rate. Even the attitudes of those who skipped breakfast were adversely affected.

The reasons given for skipping breakfast were ordinarily these: oversleeping; snacking late at night and then not being hungry for breakfast; breakfast not ready and no time to prepare it; spending too much time getting ready for school. It is improbable that the needed nourishment, except for calories, will be made up during the day if breakfast is missed. If a second meal is omitted, the lack of nourishment is that much greater.

A reason for skipping other meals is the teen-ager's busy schedule. He is often "on the go" from early morning till night with schoolwork and extracurricular activities. If a date is coming up or a party with the gang, meals are unimportant. As might be expected, girls miss more meals than boys.

Including too little milk is another fault of adolescents. Since milk is a significant source of calcium which is needed for growth, and adolescence is a period of fast growth, it is recommended that four cups be included daily. Because teen-agers frequently take less than the recommended amount of milk, their diets tend to be low in calcium. In one survey it was found that fewer than a fourth of the girls and a little more than half of the boys drank four cups of milk daily. Three fourths of the girls and 90 percent of the boys had two cups of milk a day, however. Some tend to substitute coffee for milk as they get older. In one report the drinking of coffee and tea was shown to increase from 5 percent in grades seven to nine to 15 percent in grade twelve.

Such expressions as "between-agers," "transition," "maturing" used in describing the teen years imply a period of preparation for another important role in life, that of parenthood. Although teen-age boys and girls are still in the formative years and not ready to take on the stress and responsibility of family life, many of them do. More than half of all the girls fifteen to nineteen years of age have been or are married. As a result, teen-age pregnancies are increasing. In addition, there are many unwed teen-age mothers. In 1962, 14 percent of all babies born in the United States had mothers under nineteen years of age. More than a third of these girls were under fifteen years old. In 1965 there were 7,768 babies born to ten- to fourteen-year-old mothers.

Imposing the extra stress of pregnancy on a girl still in her formative years, whose body demands a large supply of nutrients to complete its own growth, is a risk to both mother and child. The younger the mother the greater the hazard. According to the *American Journal of Obstetrics and Gynecology* teen-age pregnancies have more complications such as toxemia, prolonged labor, premature births, and cesarean sections. There is also a higher incidence of defects, abnormalities, and deaths in infants.

In *Nutrition Today,* December, 1968, Dr. Lucille Hurley states that clues from animal experiments "lead us to suspect that many birth defects may be caused by food the mother eats—or neglects to eat. . . . The younger the mother, the less likely she is to enjoy professional guidance during pregnancy and the more likely she is to commit all the nutritional sins common to teen-agers."

Teen-age girls are prone to go on diets whether they need them or not. Dr. Ruth Huenemann and her associates found in questioning about 1,000 teen-agers, that they were very figure-conscious. A typical case involves Marian, a petite high school girl. As a typical teen-age girl, she was frequently putting herself on a diet. Her family did not help the situation. Teasing remarks to the effect that her very-much overweight sister was just her size at her age, would start a frenzy of dieting. In consequence she was undernourished and anemic.

Overweight is a very real teen-age problem, however, and is frequently caused by poor nutrition. The percentage of overweight in some areas has been reported to be as high as 44 percent for girls and 29 percent for boys. Dr. Huenemann reported that only about a fourth of the girls in the study were overweight, but about half of them thought they needed to reduce.

Often "crash" reducing diets are followed to the detriment of physical well-being. They deprive the users of many needed nutrients. They tend to be followed intermittently with zeal and abandoned because of hunger. The dieter then overeats of the wrong type of food and may grow fatter. The habit of skipping meals may also contribute to gain in weight as it encourages gorging at the meals and snacking between meals.

Dr. S. L. Hammar of Seattle states that it is not uncommon for teen-agers to consume the bulk of their food in the late afternoon and evening. This "night eating syndrome" alone tends to promote overweight.

The too-plump adolescent does not necessarily eat more food. He or she may eat less than slim friends but have less activity.

Recent research at Harvard University suggests genetics as an important factor in teen-age obesity. It was found that if one parent was obese, about half of the children tended to be overweight. If both parents were overweight, 80 percent of the children were obese.

"Many cases of teen-age obesity," Dr. Felix Heald, Jr., stated in the *Journal of the American Medical Association,* "have their origin in the overweight one-year-old infant, and a large percentage of obese adolescents will remain obese as adults." Prevention is the best method of approach. To establish good food habits early in life is simpler than breaking poor ones later. Well-balanced meals, not too many calories, and physical exercise should be the pattern during the entire life.

When teen-agers realize that good nutrition assists them in reaching their goals, their eating habits improve. Dr. Ercel Eppright and her associates reported their experiences in Iowa. They found that better food habits were positively related to the knowledge of nutrition and the educational level of both parents.

Better nutrition for teen-agers has been a subject of much interest and study. How can young people be motivated to practice better eating habits? The most successful programs have been based on the needs and wants of the teen-agers themselves and have actively involved them in helping to solve their own problems.

Dr. M. E. M. Herford of England stresses that health should be part of the teaching in the schools. The school lunch offers an excellent opportunity for teaching good food habits and examples of nutritious meals. The menus can be planned by the students themselves. The fun of planning, purchasing, preparing, and serving wholesome, appetizing meals stimulates their interest in nutrition.

Another avenue is through social activities. Youth tend to idolize their peers. If popular leaders can be influenced to eat wholesome food, others will copy their habits.

To the teen-ager his appearance is most important, even though to his parents' generation his styles may not be pleasing! If you can show him the positive relationship between good food and good appearance—shiny hair, clear skin, good posture, a trim figure, and radiant health—it may be the incentive to choosing a good diet. Many teen-agers suffer from acne, for instance. They welcome help and advice when they realize that their dietary habits can do much to remedy their problem.

Your example as parents in applying principles of good nutrition is significant if you hope to help your teen-agers. Good meals, well-prepared, and attractively served at regular times, will do much to encourage good dietary habits. Make mealtime a joyous, happy occasion and your teen-ager will be better nourished. Recently on a radio program a mother recounted her experiences in inducing her teen-agers to eat nutritious meals. Breakfast was her particular concern, and she increased their participation by serving interesting and unusual dishes. She planned ahead carefully so that the meals took little more time than the previous monotonous routine ones had.

Teen-age leaders with teacher counselors have launched nutrition projects with gratifying results. In Texas a three-month project involving the schools of the area and the community—parents, home economists, physicians, teachers—created such widespread interest that the students asked for more training in choosing better balanced meals and snacks. Teachers became interested and enthusiastic about teaching good nutrition, beginning in the lower grades. Local papers and television programs carried the story to new audiences. The parents and the community became eager to learn more, and the teen-agers' food choices improved. This demonstrates the potential that exists if teen-agers are rightly motivated and guided!

In summary, the importance of teen fare cannot be overemphasized since this is a period of marked growth and maturing. A poor diet may result in years of poor health. The nutritional habits of teen-agers are closely correlated to their future well-being. An adequate diet is the best health insurance.

The teen years should be a happy time of wholesome association, stimulating work and study, and preparation for the future establishment of a home. The better your teen-agers' preparation physically, mentally, and spiritually, the greater their chances for a healthy, useful, well-adjusted adult life.

BASIC MEAL PATTERN FOR TEEN-AGERS

FOOD GROUP	SERVINGS Girl	Boy*	SUGGESTED MENU
BREAKFAST			
Vegetable—fruit high in vitamin C	1	1	Orange juice
Bread—cereal	1	2	Dry cereal Toast—butter or margarine
Protein food	1	1	Egg or protein alternate
Milk	1	1	Milk—1 cup
LUNCHEON OR SUPPER			
Protein food	1	2	Burger patties
Vegetable—fruit	1	1	Apple
rich in iron	1	1	Dates or dried fruit
Bread—cereal	2	4	Whole wheat burger buns—mayonnaise
Milk	2	2	Milk—2 cups
DINNER			
Protein food	1½	2	†Lentil Loaf
Vegetable—fruit	1	2	Potato
high in vitamin A	1	1	String beans
	1	1	†Carrot and raisin salad
Bread—cereal	1	1	†Whole wheat rolls—butter or margarine Peach cobbler
Milk	1	1	Milk—1 cup

*Boy may have larger servings.

†Recipes for these dishes can be found in the companion cookbook series to this volume, *Vegetarian Cookery*.

The Harvest Years

Some students were planning to produce a skit which featured an old lady. They decided to ask the mother of one of the students to play the old lady; but the indignant student said, "My mother isn't old!" They next approached a grandmother, and she insisted that she was not old. They had no better success with a great-grandmother. When are we old? When are the harvest years?

A sprightly seventy-eight-year-old took exception to being referred to as old, and her son asked, "Well, Mother, who is old?" She quickly retorted, "Someone ten years older than I."

In the United States old age is considered to be the years after sixty-five. Sir Stanley Davidson states that in Great Britain sixty-five to seventy-five is arbitrarily called elderly and seventy-five years and over, old. Together they are referred to as aged. Actually old age comes at different times to different individuals. Some are old at forty, and others are young at ninety.

Certain physical and mental changes suggest old age—wrinkles, gray hair, lack of vigor, fatigue, poor health, so-called degenerative diseases, osteoporosis (demineralization of the bones), slowing of mental faculties, forgetfulness, and mental and emotional anxiety.

Is there any way to postpone the aging process? How is it that some are able to reach one hundred, physically and mentally active? Is it all in the genes, as some say, or is there something we can do to delay the onset of old age? Some nineteen million Americans over sixty-five (and millions more in other countries) would like to know the answer.

It is possible to influence the aging processes and prolong health and vigor. Although one's heritage appears to be a strong determinant, there are other vital factors. "Pure air, sunlight, abstemiousness, rest, exercise, proper diet, the use of water, trust in divine power—these are the true remedies" (E. G. White, *The Ministry of Healing,* page 127) and the best health and life insurance.

"Add years to life and life to years" was a slogan of Dr. Henry C. Sherman. He emphasized not just longevity but increasing the enjoyment of life. He and other scientists have shown by decades of research that nutrition is an important factor in accomplishing this. Unfortunately we are often not much concerned until signs of age become evident or we approach retirement.

"Good nutrition in old age has its base in good nutrition in early life. . . . How can youth—the aged of tomorrow—be stirred to the realization that what they will be twenty, thirty, forty, or fifty years hence depends in large measure on the food choices they make now?" asks Dr. Pearl Swanson of Iowa State University. "How can our nutrition education programs be strengthened so that all age groups will come to view food habits in terms of the future as well as of the present?"

Dr. Charles Glen King writes, "Competence of older people is in many ways a matter of nutrition." Dr. Daniel Watson at the American Dietetic Association convention in 1967 reported some improvement in memory with adequate nutrition and suggested that nutrition has a role in intellectual functions. Dr. Tom Spies has attributed the return of more youthful attributes to people comparatively young but "old in appearance and behavior" to improvement of their diets.

Dr. Swanson points out that improving the nutrition of the aging also presents a tremendous challenge, similar to that involving teenagers and nutrition. "How can they [the aging] be convinced that nutrition plays an important part in their lives, that it influences the way they think and act and feel? . . . Adequate nutrition may result in lengthening of the lifespan, positive accomplishments, greater freedom from disease, increased enjoyment of living," she says.

Bone, muscle, blood, brain, and nerve tissues are daily being replaced by the food we eat. In later years there may be decrease in the secretion of the digestive juices, lessened peristalsis, poor absorption and utilization of nutrients. These years have no growth requirement; but because there is tissue breakdown and wasting, ample protein is essential. About one fourth of the daily protein requirement will be supplied by one pint of milk. There is sometimes a tendency to restrict or avoid milk as we get older. This is poor practice in most cases, since milk not only supplies good protein but is the best source of calcium. We do not outgrow the need of calcium or other minerals and vitamins, and they should be in adequate supply. There is some evidence that a low intake of calcium is a contributing factor to osteoporosis.

Some surveys have found protein, calcium, and vitamins C and A and the B-complex most often lacking in the diet of older persons. In a study in Rochester, New York, of 283 persons with an average age of seventy-two, one fourth of the diets were poor, and less than half were good. A third of the group were overweight. In 695 older persons in an Iowa study, only one in twenty was choosing a nutritionally adequate diet, more than one third were deficient in protein, nearly two thirds in vitamins A and C, and more than three fourths in calcium. There was a tendency reported in one survey for older persons to increase the use of bread and cereals, as well as of harmful sweets and desserts.

Calories should be reduced as we get older to correspond to lessened activity. Use a lower percentage of carbohydrate, especially sweets and desserts. Avoid "empty calories." In America the usual amount of fat in the diet is about 40 percent of the calories. This should be reduced to 20 to 30 percent, largely of unsaturated fats. It has been suggested that the daily caloric intake be 1,600 to 1,800 for women and 2,000 to 2,200 for men. A vitamin and mineral supplement is frequently prescribed.

The basic requirements remain practically the same throughout adult life except for calories and individual limitations. Include daily:

Milk—two cups or more, used as a drink, in soups, or in combination with other foods.

Proteins—two or more servings of such foods as cottage cheese or other mild cheese, eggs, nuts, legumes (peas, beans, lentils, et cetera), and gluten and nut preparations.

Vegetables and fruits—four or more servings:

Dark green or deep yellow vegetable (at least 4 times weekly).

Raw vegetable salad, if tolerated.

Potatoes and a variety of other vegetables.
Citrus fruit, tomatoes, or other good sources of vitamin C.
A liberal use of a wide variety of other fruits.

Cereals and breads—whole grain (or enriched), 4 servings.

Other foods—fats and simple natural sweets to round out the diet.

When there is a tendency to gain weight, use skim milk and less starches, sweets, and fats. If additional calories are needed, more of the foods listed above or such high calorie foods as avocado, olives, dates, and dried fruits may be added.

Some Suggested Menus

BREAKFAST	**BREAKFAST**	**BREAKFAST**
Grapefruit 1 egg 1 slice buttered toast Cereal coffee	Orange juice Apple sauce 2 slices toast Peanut butter Postum made with milk	Mixed fruit juice Oatmeal, milk 1 slice buttered toast Cocoa
DINNER	**DINNER**	**DINNER**
†Soyameat Casserole Green beans Carrot salad Roll, butter or margarine Milk Ice cream	†Glutenburger loaf Baked potato, sour cream and chives Spinach, lemon Bread, butter or margarine Apricot nectar Tapioca pudding	Baked macaroni and cheese Buttered broccoli Sliced tomato Bread, butter or margarine Buttermilk Filled cookie
SUPPER OR LUNCH	**SUPPER OR LUNCH**	**SUPPER OR LUNCH**
Pineapple and cottage cheese salad Tomato-avocado sandwich Hot ovaltine	Cream of vegetable soup Fruit salad Buttered toast Milk	Creamed split peas on toast Sliced peaches Milk

Regularity is important. Meals may need to be spaced with longer intervals between. Sometimes smaller and more frequent meals may be required. Heavy meals and foods difficult to digest should be avoided.

When constipation is a problem, drink more water (especially be-

†Recipes for these dishes can be found in the companion cookbook series to this volume, *Vegetarian Cookery*.

fore breakfast) and use fruits, vegetables, and juices freely. Light exercise such as a daily walk is beneficial and helps to stimulate the appetite and improves the health in general.

Securing an adequate diet when one is advanced in years is not always simple. Shopping for groceries or even the effort of preparing a meal is sometimes beyond one's strength. Especially is this true for the person bent with arthritis, one who is racked with pain or short of breath, one with heart trouble or other disabilities. Add to this the problems of finance, of living and eating alone, of no teeth or ill-fitting dentures, of previously established food habits and patterns and food intolerances or prejudices, and it is not difficult to see why malnutrition is common in the harvest years.

Poor appetite frequently plagues the elderly. This may be due to lack of exercise and fresh air, slower body functions, or difficulty in eating resulting from poor teeth or dentures; but too often it is related to loneliness, heartache, anxiety, and worry.

Take the case of Mr. Heeber. He had filled the same important position in a college for forty years. He had excellent health and in all the years had lost very few days due to illness. His life centered around his work and his home. When he neared seventy, he was retired. His wife had died, and his children had married. Suddenly his whole life pattern was disrupted. He was lost and desperately lonely. He had no appetite, lost weight, and rapidly deteriorated physically and mentally.

Mrs. Victor was a homebody and a superior cook whose life centered in her husband and children. After her children left home and her husband died, she became a hospital volunteer, visited and helped those in need, and took an interest in community affairs. She had made a good adjustment and all went well until she became crippled with arthritis and entered a rest home. Here the food was nourishing but vastly different from her own good cooking. She could not get about and was lonely. But she had a firm trust in God and prayed that He would help her to find those she could help and encourage. She began counting her blessings, and her cheerful philosophy of life became an inspiration to many.

These cases could be multiplied by the thousands, perhaps millions. Adding years to life and life to years involves more than providing good nutrition. As Dr. Wendell Griffith once stated, "Nutrition cannot be separated easily from economic, medical, psychological, and social factors."

There is no standard formula for growing old creatively and graciously. The mature years are harvesttime when the results of a lifetime are reaped. To live a longer, more vigorous and abundant life, observe the following arithmetic: *Subtract* harmful practices and any intemperances; *divide* your calories by your exercise; *add* nutritious foods, pure water, fresh air and sunlight, mild activity, adequate rest, a sense of humor, kind thoughts of others, and calm trust in God. As you do this you will *multiply* health and vigor, and your enjoyment of life will increase. "A merry heart doeth good like a medicine," so *count* your blessings and be thankful.